No Expiration Dates

No Expiration Dates

A Cancer Patient's Strategies for Survival

Leon Weisman

iUniverse, Inc.

New York   Bloomington

No Expiration Dates
A Cancer Patient's Strategies for Survival

The views expressed in this work are solely those of the author and do not necessarily reflect the views of the publisher, and the publisher hereby disclaims any responsibility for them.

iUniverse books may be ordered through booksellers or by contacting:

iUniverse
1663 Liberty Drive
Bloomington, IN 47403
www.iuniverse.com
1-800-Authors (1-800-288-4677)

Because of the dynamic nature of the Internet, any Web addresses or links contained in this book may have changed since publication and may no longer be valid. The views expressed in this work are solely those of the author and do not necessarily reflect the views of the publisher, and the publisher hereby disclaims any responsibility for them.

ISBN: 978-1-4401-6868-0 (pbk)
ISBN: 978-1-4401-6869-7 (cloth)
ISBN: 978-1-4401-6870-3 (ebk)

Library of Congress Control Number: 2009935493

Printed in the United States of America

iUniverse rev. date: 9/21/2009

Illustrations by Marlene Weisman-Abadi

Contents

About this Book   ix

Acknowledgments   xi

Introduction   xiii

1. Hospitals, Physicians, and Hospital Time   1
2. Sharing the News   7
3. Chemo World   11
4. No Expiration Dates   15
5. Living with Fatigue   19
6. Embracing the Insignificant   25
7. Moving beyond Grief   29
8. Searching for the Truth   33
9. Funny Bones   37
10. Higher-Level Thinking   41
11. Mothers with Cancer   49
12. Creating Comfort Zones   57
13. The Vocabulary of Cancer   61
14. Death Re-viewed   65
15. The Arms of Morpheus   69
16. The Appearance of Men   73
17. The Difficult Patient   77
18. Directed Speech   81
19. Mending Wall   85
20. Controlling Control   91

21. Unfulfilled Dreams   97
22. Releasing Purse Strings   105
23. Attitude Adjustment   111
Resource Guide   117
Bibliography   121
Afterword   123

Yesterday is experience. Tomorrow is hope.
Today is getting from one to the other as best we can.
—John M. Henry

About this Book

It has been said that the longest journey starts with a single step. Many adventurers and explorers take that first step with a manual for survival tucked in their backpacks.

In similar fashion, *No Expiration Dates* is a memoir of discovery—a blueprint for survival for people who are traveling a difficult and precarious route. For the cancer patient, staying alive is a full-time chore. This book of suggestions, strategies, and plans of action can be an invaluable aid in formulating a new way of life.

For relatives and friends, I have provided valuable insights to foster greater compassion for those living with cancer. For the general public, the book is a passport to a new world—an excursion into the realm of quiet desperation.

I have organized this book in a systematic fashion, featuring three distinct components:

- An initial quote is a springboard into the chapter. This quote provides foresight and forethought for the reader by providing a "mental set."
- The text of the chapter follows, with a compilation of observations, suggestions, and problems experienced by the author—a cancer patient himself.
- Each chapter concludes with a series of "end quotes" designed to stimulate the reader's thoughts. The culmination of the chapter is enhanced by these perceptive quotes, whose ideas I have incorporated into the chapter. Note that the assemblage of the chapters is consistent. The components remain the same to facilitate familiarity through repetition. This makes for easier reading.

No Expiration Dates is a memoir of hope and survival. Climbing Mount Everest or traversing the Serengetti may not be in your plans right now. However, you may currently have your own version of Mount Everest to scale, and reaching the summit is within your grasp.

A resource guide listing the telephone numbers and Internet addresses for thirty-five cancer-related organizations is included for additional support services.

This is a book of hope. Read it with an eye on the horizon.

Acknowledgments

I wish to express my gratitude to the entire cancer care team and the office staff of the Queens-Long Island Medical Group in Woodbury and Hicksville, New York.

To my beautiful and courageous wife, Sylvia, whose love and support breathes life into my soul, I am indebted beyond words.

To my devoted son, Steven, and his wife, Lauren, and to my dear daughter, Marlene, and her husband, Michael, I express gratitude of mountainous proportions.

My precious grandchildren, Andrew and Adam, thank you for your hugs and kisses.

I pay special thanks to my cousins Ron and Marjorie Miller and Sid and Marilyn Buchman for their deep concern and commitment to my recovery.

Special recognition must be afforded to my dear friends Sheila Thau, Alan Bergstein and Marjorie Bitson, Marilyn and Joe Greene, Sunny and Jules Organ, and Bernard and Hortense Chenkin, who have shown their love and support beyond anything I could expect.

And to Dr. Bruce and Gloria Dorman, please accept my gratitude for being dedicated neighbors.

Introduction

You can never plan the future by the past.

—*Edmund Burke*

The sleek Lear air ambulance sliced through the fragrant evening skies blanketing the Boca Raton Airport, ferrying a seventy-five-year-old lung cancer patient to North Shore University Hospital in Manhasset, New York.

Accompanied by my wife, Sylvia; two paramedics; and two pilots, the awesome power of the jet engines strained the gurney straps and put pressure on the mass nestled in my right lung.

Cruising altitude was reached, and monitoring equipment kept a continuous flow of my vital signs.

Touchdown occurred at midnight, with the air ambulance landing safely at Republic Airfield in Farmingdale, New York. A synchronized team of EMTs processed the transfer of Sylvia and myself from plane to ground ambulance.

The winter's chill seared my face as I was exposed to the new climate from which we sought escape thirty days ago.

Heading toward North Shore University Hospital, the pulsating red and white emergency lights encountered a falling snow. "From balmy to stormy," I thought. "Perhaps it is a metaphor for my uncertain future."

UNCERTAINTY

I have never smoked. My contact with caustic substances has been minimal—restricted to summer foliage and crab grass sprays.

On January 1, 2007, my routine flight to Miami developed nightmarish characteristics. Due to engine complications, passengers had to endure a three-hour tarmac delay, with seat restrictions. This episode could have been responsible for releasing pulmonary embolisms in both legs, which began their northern trek to my lungs.

We had begun our vacation with a delightful cruise that departed from Miami on January 2. The pristine waters and azure skies of the Caribbean held little portent of what lay ahead. Our ten-day cruise ended on a high: no signs of physical distress, and a tolerable northern ride on I-95 to Deerfield Beach in a comfortable rental auto.

Sylvia and I planned to stay at our favorite resort from January 12 to January 23, flying back to New York on Tuesday, January 24.

I was eager to return to prepare for the spring semester at Queensborough Community College and Nassau Community College—in Bayside, Queens, and Garden City, Long Island, respectively. I am an adjunct professor at both colleges.

The Florida vacation had become an annual ritual to renew old friendships with ex-New Yorkers who'd fled the ravages of winter for the embrace of Florida sun. I'd created a schedule to ensure adequate visiting time for relatives and friends.

The pièce de résistance was to be a salmon dinner at the Boca Raton home of my dear friends Alan and Marjorie. As I penciled in that Sunday dinner, little did I realize the nature of the event that was to occur at the dinner's conclusion.

Life was good! Seven days of radiant sun, no rain, cool breezes, and a rented Chevy Impala performing admirably.

During my years as a visitor to Deerfield Beach, I'd established the routine of an evening stroll on the pebbly paved path snaking along the Atlantic shoreline. Markers embedded in the walkway measure out the distance a walker has achieved. I have always been an accomplished walker!

Shortly after my usual stroll commenced on Friday, January 19, I was seized with belabored breathing, chest pain, and oxygen deprivation. Struggling to stay erect, I sat on one of the benches facing the churning Atlantic surf. My regular breathing resumed, and I returned to my hotel.

For some inexplicable reason, I did not share the experience with Sylvia. The next day was uneventful, with no symptoms reoccurring—until that evening.

My stroll along the beach on the next evening, January 20, produced the same symptoms as the previous evening. I rested and returned to the hotel with nary a word to my wife about what was developing.

As planned, the next evening we arrived at the Boca home of our gracious hosts, Marjorie and Alan. After a delicious meal, Alan volunteered to accompany Sylvia and me to the parking lot, where my Impala waited in a guest space.

As the elevator reached the ground floor, I experienced a full-scale attack of belabored breathing, chest pain, and gasps for air. Alan's cell phone came into immediate use, and the Boca Raton Fire-Rescue Services arrived in moments.

Alan ... had saved ... my life.

My life. Ebbing. Fading. Was it to end here inside an ambulance?

"We're losing him!" I recall hearing.

How appropriate for Florida to wash me away to distant shores.

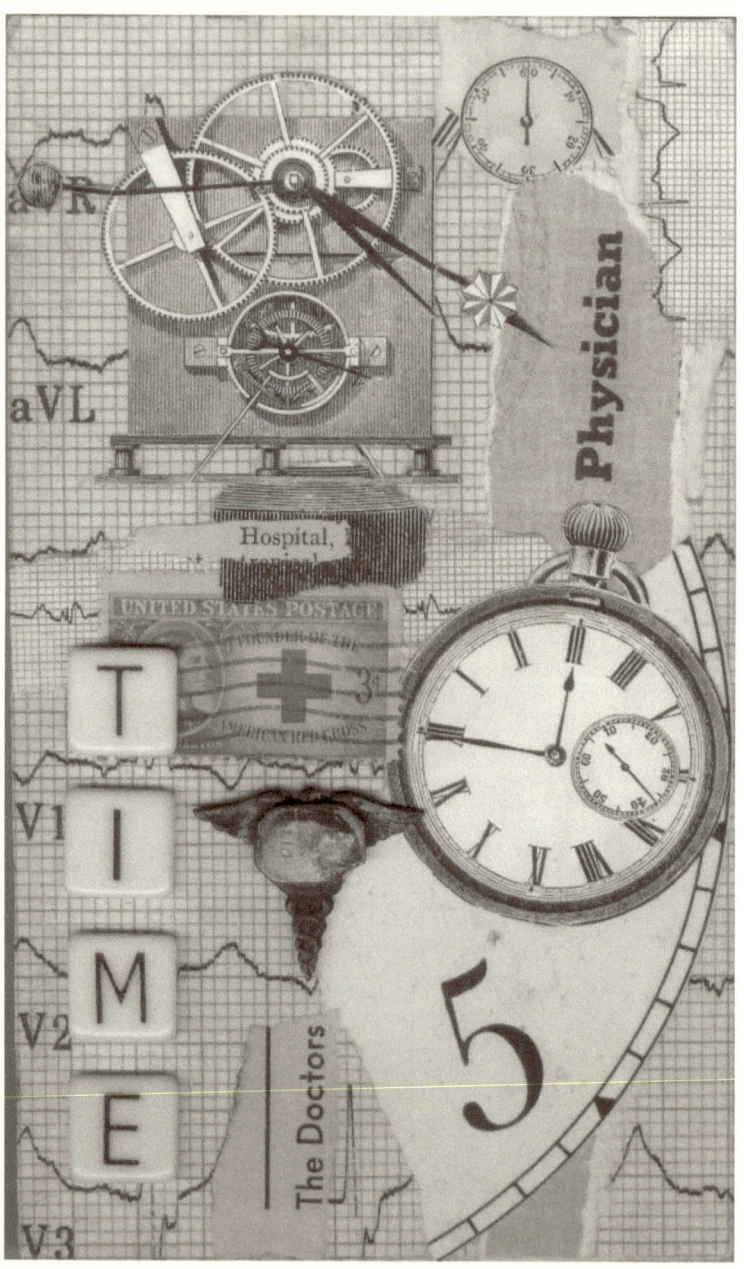

Chapter One

Hospitals, Physicians, and Hospital Time

Nature, time and patience are the three great
physicians.

—*Unknown*

HOSPITALS

Located in the beautiful city of Boca Raton, the community hospital is situated northwest of Deerfield Beach.

The hospital's façade is a medical oxymoron. Palm trees, waterfalls, and a lake landscaped with pink tropical foliage contrast sharply with the vast number of snowbirds who become ill on their southern retreat and seek medical attention within its tropical charm.

A piano player in the lobby greets visitors to the strains of Stravinsky. Sculptures line the corridors, amidst bronze plaques recording the philanthropic gestures of concerned residents. We don't usually think of hospitals as "user-friendly." However, I watched a closed-circuit bingo game presided over by a senior volunteer who awarded prizes to winners.

Winners in a hospital—an interesting twist of fate.

A team of well-tanned medical experts spoke in guarded tones and introduced the specter of lung cancer. All agreed, however, that biopsies must be performed as soon as I returned home.

Two days after my emergency admittance to the hospital, my son, Steven, and his darling wife, Lauren, arrived in Boca Raton from their home in Holbrook, New York. This action was greatly appreciated since Steven is an administrator at Stony Brook University Hospital on Long Island. His knowledge of hospital operation provided a high degree of assurance. Steven was in constant communication with his sister, Marlene Weisman-Abadi; her husband, Michael; and seven-year-old Adam.

Steven's sixteen-year-old son, Andrew, arranged to board at a friend's house; and Diane and Bernard Lebowitz, Steven's in-laws, kindly volunteered to care for Shea, their playful West Highland Terrier.

The urgency for immediate internal exploration resulted in my leaving Boca Raton Community Hospital on the evening of Monday, January 29, via air ambulance, for my Long Island hospital.

Situated on Community Drive in Manhasset, New York, North Shore University Hospital fulfills its theme of "setting the standard for medical care." With prompt concern, a medical team was assembled. The attending physician was compassionate and dependable. The oncologist exuded confidence in his planning. The pulmonologist performed the biopsy with precision. A resident physician buoyed my spirits when depression set in. A lanky intern was apologetic when he delivered distressing news.

The hospital housed every conceivable device to delve into the recesses of my body. Their staff of pathologists and radiologists issued their reports with dispatch.

In a display of remarkable devotion, my daughter, Marlene, spent one week in my hospital room, sleeping on a lounge chair. My wife, Sylvia, accompanied her during daytime hours but returned home in the evenings. Steven, Marlene, and Lauren performed Herculean tasks of contacting insurance companies, coordinating hospital activities, and attending to dietary issues.

In addition to attending to my needs, Marlene, Steven, and Lauren provided support and attention for Sylvia, who endures the debilitating pain of lumbar stenosis and osteoarthritis.

PHYSICIANS

A hospital is a cloister of medical scholars. Speaking in strange tongues, they use words meant to explain your condition. The words fly at you as each "ologist" presents his or her findings in measured gaits.

Styles vary. The physician who speaks in whispers reassures his patient by employing an aura of confidence. The doctor who emotes resoundingly projects an image of a living textbook. Some doctors resemble professors, while others portray a picture of "dress-down" casual.

The speed at which physicians can appear at your bedside is impressive. Unannounced, they float in and out, making their daily rounds.

In many respects, doctors resemble judges. They weigh the evidence, consider the alternatives, and offer acquittal, probation, or sentencing.

HOSPITAL TIME

Is there a definition of time?

Railroad time, airport time, and TV time are examples of precise time and dependability.

The hospital patient enters a befuddling dimension known as "hospital time." Schedules are mere suggestions, appointments are fluid, and daytime and nighttime have lost their power of partition. The work schedules of physicians and hospital staff utilize a twenty-four-hour clock.

The volume of patients awaiting X-rays, CAT and PET scans, and ultrasound tests causes a backup of gurneys, wheelchairs, and hospital beds. Similar to the stacking of airplanes awaiting landing rights at major airports, patients await their turn in silent agony.

When your turn is announced, you enter a room of nuclear-age furnishings—equipment of exploration beyond imagination. With great concern, compassionate technicians insert patients in the devices.

Radiologists and pathologists remain unseen and monitor the "pictures" with eyes entrusted to interpreting secrets entombed within the body.

You issue a sigh of relief when you are dismissed and permitted to return to the comfort of your hospital room. Time will stand still. The hands of hospital clocks move in slow motion.

END QUOTES

Everything happens to everybody sooner or later if there is time enough.

—George Bernard Shaw

Time is the valuable thing a person can spend.

—Theophrastus

The very first requirement in a hospital is that it should do the sick no harm.

—Florence Nightingale

There are some remedies worse than the disease.

—Publilius Syrus

Don't defy the diagnosis, try to defy the verdict.

—Norman Cousins

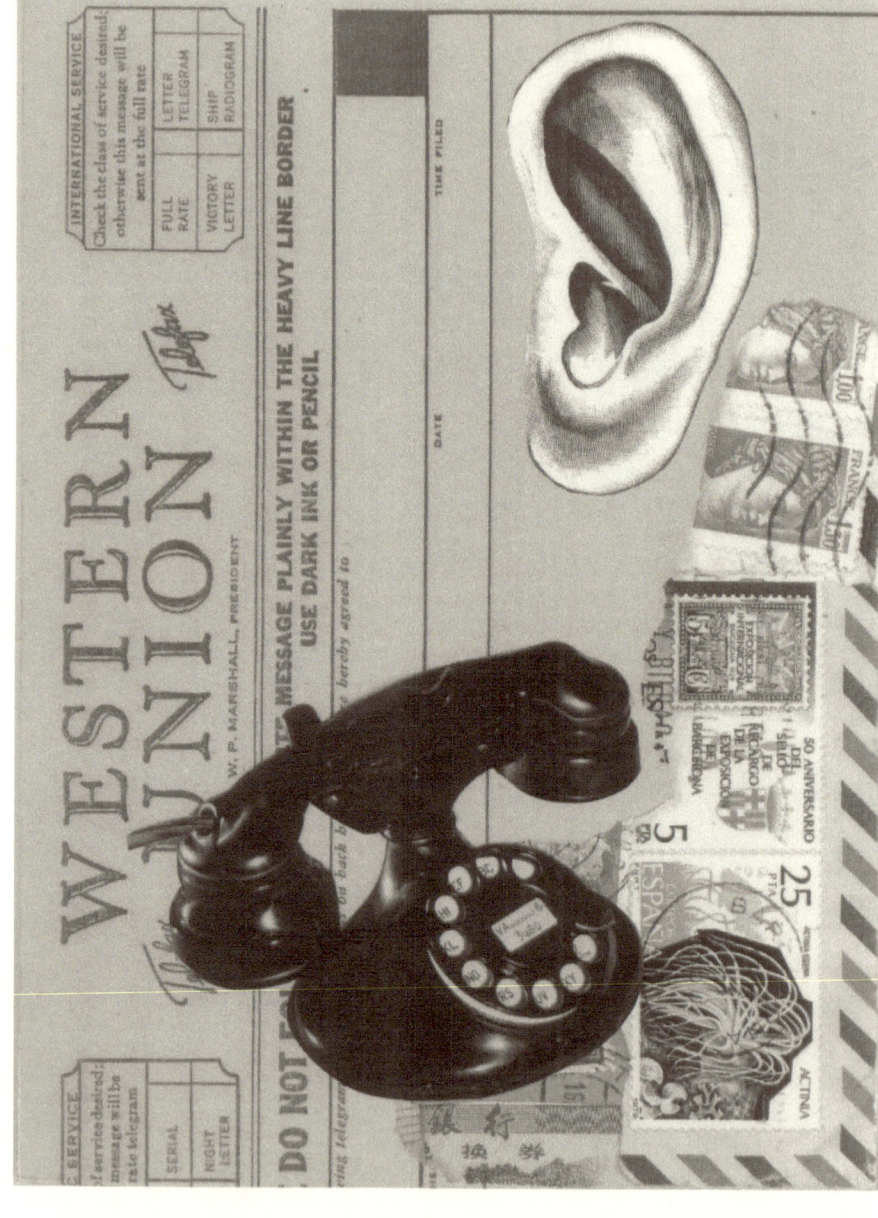

Chapter Two

Sharing the News

News travels fast. Bad news travels faster.
—Unknown

Some linguists claim *news* is an acronym for north, east, west, and south—referring to the points of the compass. Others prefer the more conservative definition of "a recent occurrence; of significant importance—an event worthwhile of comment."

Whatever definition you prefer, there exists a situation where relatives, friends, and colleagues need to be informed of your illness.

There was a time when the word "cancer" was unutterable. It was referred to as the "Big C," with people unable to say the word for fear of impending consequences. Times have changed. Restrictions are relaxed, and people are more open to its acceptance.

It will be difficult to keep your illness a secret. Cancer patients become topics of conversation: causes célèbres.

Conversations regarding your situation often start with three familiar words: "Have you heard …?"

Friends, relatives, and colleagues may not see you at familiar haunts. Your appearance may have changed from loss of hair and weight. Walking may be impaired by loss of balance. How long can you hide the truth from them?

To tell or not to tell is a decision you must make. My decision was to share the news. I was greeted by a series of comments from callers talking with muffled sobs:

- Are you sure?
- How bad is it?
- What is the prognosis?
- How do they know?
- But you never smoked!

Conversations ended in several ways: abruptly, with the caller unable to continue; sympathetically, with the caller offering assurance of recovery; and defiantly, with the caller challenging a higher authority for creating such a catastrophic situation.

For those who choose an indirect communication, e-mail may suffice. However, personal contact is the best way to conduct your mission.

Although I have found all recipients of the news of my lung cancer to be quite compassionate, it would not surprise me that there are hard-liners out there. "Sympathy," they may think, "can be found in the dictionary between *symmetry* and *symphony*." However, I believe this reaction is an exception.

In kindergarten, we learn that *sharing is caring.* Devoted relatives, friends of many years, and workaday colleagues deserve to know. Your pain will be lessened when you share it with many.

Spouses and marriage partners deserve special consideration. Their lives may be directly affected. Keeping them abreast of dates for treatments, blood tests, infusions, and injections is vital. A calendar is an excellent data-keeping device.

Can the onset of cancer affect a marriage or a relationship? Probably. Tensions, uncertainty, schedules, and bills are not conducive to fostering happy times. Both sides must strive to reduce these difficult times.

Bill Cosby said, "The heart of marriage is memories." Don't disregard the past. Recall the good times and build on the love, trust, and partnership of the pre-illness days.

END QUOTES

It is better to know some of the questions than all of the answers.

—James Thurber

Sticks and stones may break our bones, but words will break our hearts.

—Robert Fulghum

The less you talk, the more you're listened to.

—Abigail Van Buren

The two words "information" and "communication" are often used interchangeably, but they signify quite different things. Information is giving out, communication is getting through.

—Sidney J. Harris

News is the same old thing—only happening to different people.

—Unknown

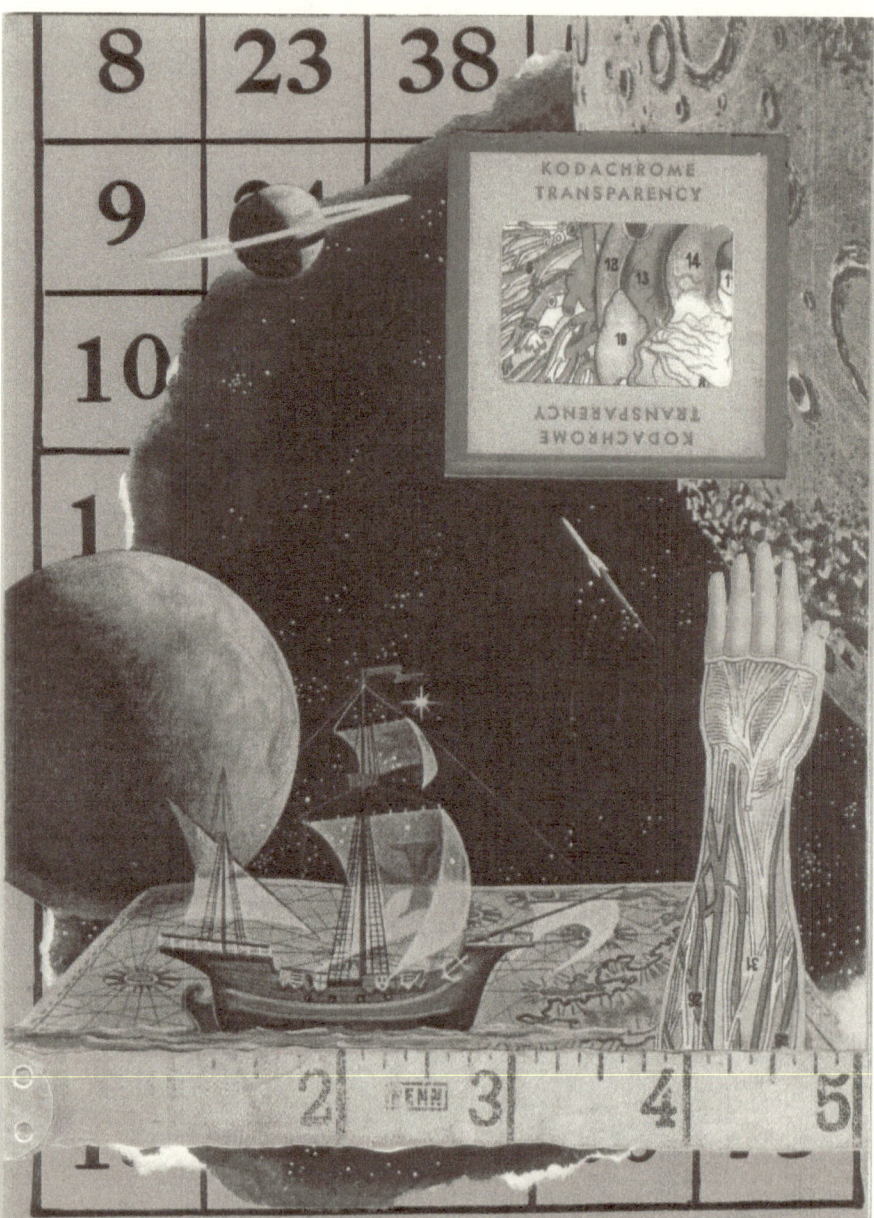

Chapter Three

Chemo World

You're never a loser, until you quit trying.
—*Mike Ditka*

The uninitiated may wonder where chemotherapy takes place. The answer will vary according to the physical layout of the facility. Larger communal areas, individual booths containing a single "lounger," or semi-private spaces where you have one partner are the most common.

My experiences with countless chemotherapy sessions have been in a communal area containing seven reclining chairs with footrests. For most sessions, all seven chairs are occupied. At my center, faux leather in gray, brown, and azure complement the yellow walls, with nary two feet of space separating each chair. Six-foot metal poles held erect by star-shaped pedestals support plastic bags containing chemo protocols.

Magazines are present in a rack attached to the wall, and a supply of used paperbacks lines the windowsill.

Two television sets feed a continuous stream of cable news into the refrigerated air.

Brightly clad nurses hover among the patients in response to the beeping of pumps signaling stoppage of flow into the veins of the recipients. Pumps are quickly reset, and the chemotherapy continues its therapeutic passage.

Patients vary in their activities during chemo sessions, which may last up to five hours.

Snacks appear from tote bags containing cookies, crackers, chips, or candy bars. I recall the smell of a meat sandwich wafting through the chemo sanctuary as one patient munched away, oblivious to the serums coursing through his veins.

After my first unfortunate experience of purging during a chemo session, I made a practice of keeping a plastic bag in my pocket to collect any food reflexively seeking an exit.

To be forewarned is to be forearmed. Chemotherapy requires that a person prepare for surprises. Prepare for the worst but expect the best.

Some cancer patients refuse chemotherapy. Indeed, it is a very significant decision—quite serious and critical. Consider the consequences, your loved ones, and its importance to your recovery. In my situation, refusal was never an option.

END QUOTES

Illness is not something a person has, it's another way of being.

—Jonathan Miller

When the going gets tough, the tough get going.

—Joseph P. Kennedy

Words of comfort, skillfully administered, are the oldest therapy known to man.

—Louis Nizer

Correction does much, but encouragement does more.

—Wolfgang Von Geothe

The fragrance always stays in the hand that gives the rose.

—Hada Bejar

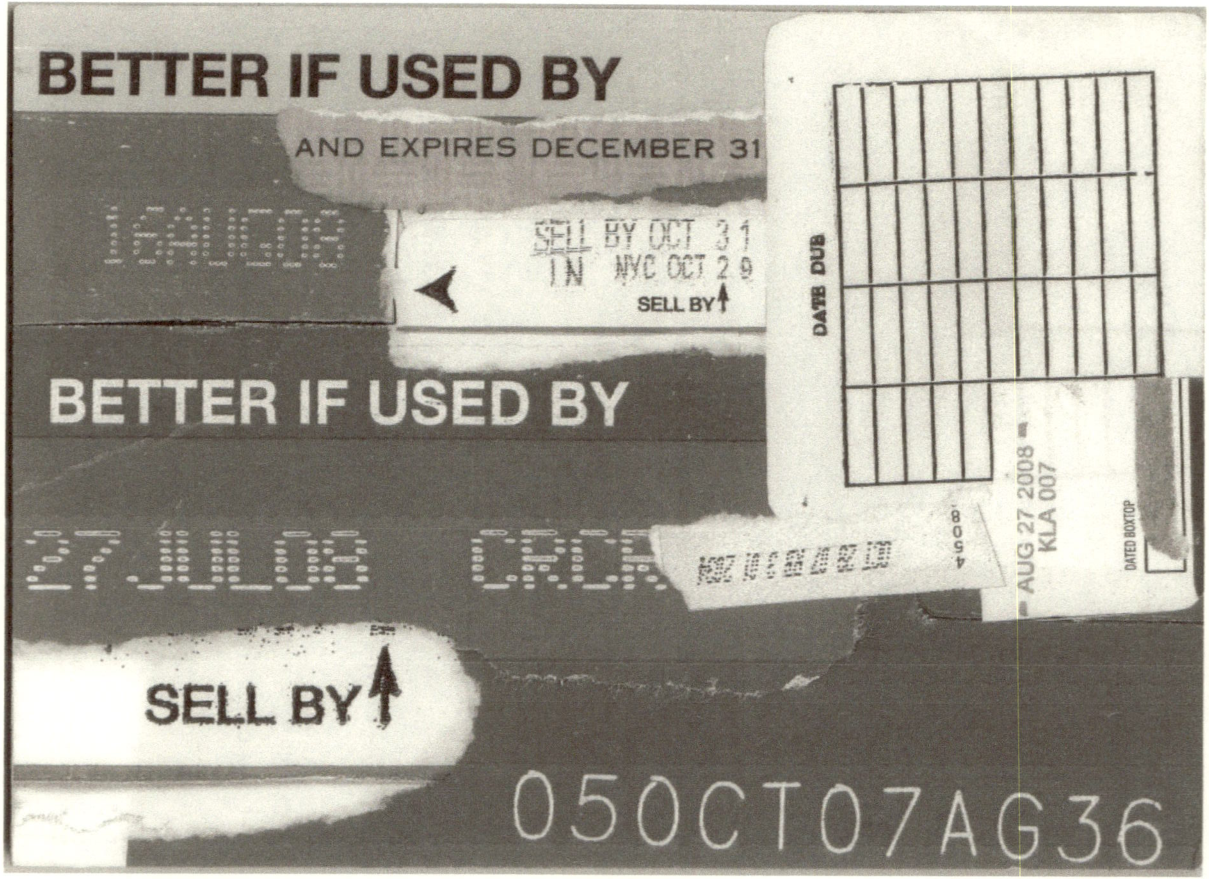
BETTER IF USED BY
AND EXPIRES DECEMBER 31
SELL BY OCT 31
IN NYC OCT 29
SELL BY
DATE DUE
BETTER IF USED BY
27JUL08
AUG 27 2008
KLA 007
DATED BOXTOP
SELL BY
05OCT07AG36

Chapter Four

No Expiration Dates

Oh, never say that you have reached the very end,
though leaden skies a bitter future may portend.
—*Hirsch Glick*

Examine your body carefully. Explore its crevasses, nooks, crannies, and recesses.

Can you find an expiration date?

Hardly.

An exploration of your cupboard or refrigerator will reveal a multitude of products stamped with expiration dates. These dates protect the consumer by predicting the product's shelf life and preventing bacteria from accumulating.

Cancer patients do *not* have expiration dates. Expiration is the nemesis of hope. Expiration is an absolute term bearing no significance for individual consideration.

Why, then, do doctors feel incumbent upon them to pronounce expiration dates on many of their patients? Unfortunately, I was one of them. The shock is devastating and life altering. It argues a "getting-your-house-in-order" attitude, and your Book of Life becomes an instant short story. To hear the words of a death sentence is unimaginable. Its stunning effect is paralytic.

How can the recipient of an expiration date by an insensitive physician recover from the initial shock? Your strength rests within the word itself:

E X P I <u>R</u> A T I O N

The *pir* is found in "s<u>pir</u>it," "ins<u>pir</u>e," and "res<u>pir</u>ation"—meaning vitality, breathing, and hope. Look within yourself as well as at the word itself. Derive strength to obliterate any date impregnated on your mind. Statistically they are meaningless, psychologically they are destructive, and intellectually they are spurious.

Removing an expiration date is a gesture of freedom. Renewal of life forces, eyes focused on the future, and sleep-laden nights may result from this change. An expiration date is exclusionary. The cancer patient is cast into a special class of "temporary occupants," whose presence is no longer counted. Cancer patients are very much part of the population—thriving, working, and striving to maintain a normal lifestyle.

In many societies, lepers were outcasts. Fear, mysticism, and fences shut out these people. In today's world, the cancer patient remains an integral part of the fabric of our society.

Coupons and medicines have expiration dates—a sure sign of eventual discard. Terminated and finished, their journey is completed.

For many cancer patients, their journey has just begun.

END QUOTES

I am the master of my fate. I am the captain of my soul.
—W. E. Henley

I never think of the future. It comes soon enough.
—Albert Einstein

You don't get to choose how you're going to die. Or when. You can only decide how you're going to live.
—Joan Baez

Dying is a very dull, dreary affair. And my advice to you is to have nothing whatever to do with it.
—W. Somerset Maugham

Old age is having too much room in the house and not enough room in the medicine cabinet.
—Orben's Current Comedy

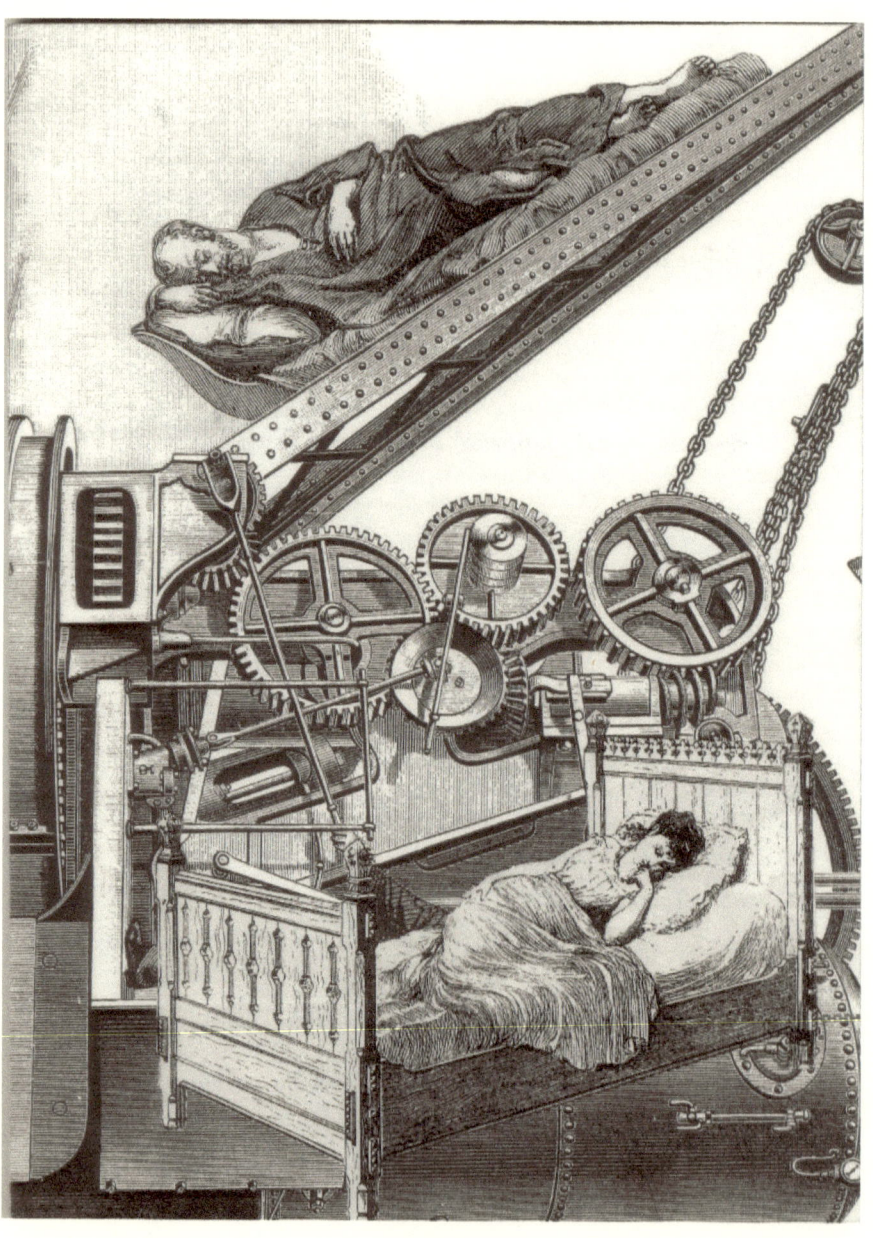

Chapter Five

Living with Fatigue

There is moderation in everything.

—Horace

An overwhelming number of cancer patients experience fatigue. Loss of strength, lack of vitality, and general malaise quite frequently occur because of chemotherapy and diminishing red blood cells.

This shutdown of the body's power plant encourages your partnership with Morpheus. An overhaul of the routines practiced prior to the disease is mandatory. Your lifestyle will be drastically affected, especially in the area of daily routines.

Giving up control of your daily activities is not an easy objective. This may require curtailing activities, slower pacing, and resetting your biological clock. Frequent naps and rest periods may help to renew and refresh tired muscles.

PEAK PERIODS

Anticipate fatigue shortly after chemo sessions. My experience indicates a two-to-three- day weakness post-chemo. Go easy. Listen to your body. It will provide you with valuable information pertinent to the revitalization of your strength. Avoid overtaxing your resources; do not let your goals exceed your grasp during this hiatus.

ACTIVITIES

Differentiate between mental and physical fatigue. Both may be present. In that case, a cessation of all activities may be in order. However, if your mental state is alert and responsive, many daily routines can be performed:

- Accept telephone calls from relatives and friends.
- Encourage short visits from supporters.
- Read a minimum of favorite material.
- Work on bills and claims.
- Take a nap.
- Pursue an avocation or area of interest from pre-illness days.
- Discover a new area of interest that can be enlightening but does not require excessive physical activity.
- Your personal computer offers many opportunities to contact outside agencies regarding your illness.
- Television can be a welcome respite offering a wide variety of entertainment or discussions of social interest.
- Music has a soporific effect on jangled nerves. The soothing strains of popular or classical music may alleviate anxiety and tension. If country, rock, or rhythm and blues is more to your taste, schedule a period of listening at your convenience.

SNACKING

Many cancer patients experience weight loss. You may wish to take steps to combat weight loss by frequent snacking. A plethora of snacks is available in an infinite number of varieties, sizes, and tastes. Snacks have the potential to fortify energy, assuage hunger, and provide comfort.

RESCHEDULING

A fatigued state will probably require a modification and reorganization of daily routines. Some of these routines may have been practiced for many years prior to the onset of the illness.

This "rescheduling" will affect your lifestyle as well as the understanding of your condition by friends and relatives.

Days may end earlier. Bedtimes change. Meals may be adjusted to complement your new bedtime. Your new schedules may awaken friends and relatives to the realization that cancer brings inevitable adjustments. Accepting your new schedule will often present difficulties to those who see change as a disturbing influence. Rise above that. Give up your control and go with the flow.

LOSS OF BALANCE

On two occasions, I have experienced a loss of balance, resulting in noninjurious falls. To counter this, I used a cane as a stabilizer.

Why this was occurring is puzzling to me. However, I have heard similar complaints from fellow patients. Walking is a bit more precarious, with measured gaits and a wary eye out for curbstones, gratings, and railings.

Walking is still considered a good exercise, although precautions must take place. Thoreau said, "An early morning walk is a blessing for the whole day." Be careful and alert to dangers when you walk and watch the world go by.

APPLIANCES

A plastic shower chair is a valuable asset to maintain your cleanliness. If fatigue is present, you may sit while showering, and the result is refreshing. I have one in my shower, and it is quite effective.

The bathroom toilet can be equipped with guardrails. The kit can be ordered commercially and assembled easily. I have one in my bathroom, and it facilitates toilet usage.

A wheelchair can be a valuable asset for covering larger areas such as shopping malls or super-sized stores. Most insurance policies will cover the rental cost.

There is no loss of dignity when using a wheelchair. I keep one in my garage and actually enjoy being transported by a "pusher." People are respectful, children see you at the same height, and smiles occur more frequently from strangers.

CANES AND WALKERS

Canes and walkers are valuable adjuncts for walking. They both complement balance, aid fatigue, and provide a "third leg." My cane is adjustable, spiffy looking, and made of metal. I also use it to move or recover objects when I am sitting.

I am convinced that a cane is man's best friend. I have adapted my cane for "extracurricular" activities. It is an extension of my arm for retrieval and moving of objects. In addition, I use my cane for top shelves, under-the-bed items, and as a door opener. There have been times when my cane has shut off an air conditioner by depressing the OFF button. Overall, canes and walkers have a prominent position in combating fatigue.

END QUOTES

Man is harder than iron, stronger than stone and more fragile than a rose.

—Turkish proverb

There is nothing stronger in the world than gentleness.

—Han Suyin

Fall seven times, stand up eight.

—Japanese proverb

Laziness is nothing more than resting before you get tired.

—Jules Renard

In the confrontation between the stream and the rock, the stream always wins—not through strength but by perseverance.

—H. Jackson Brown

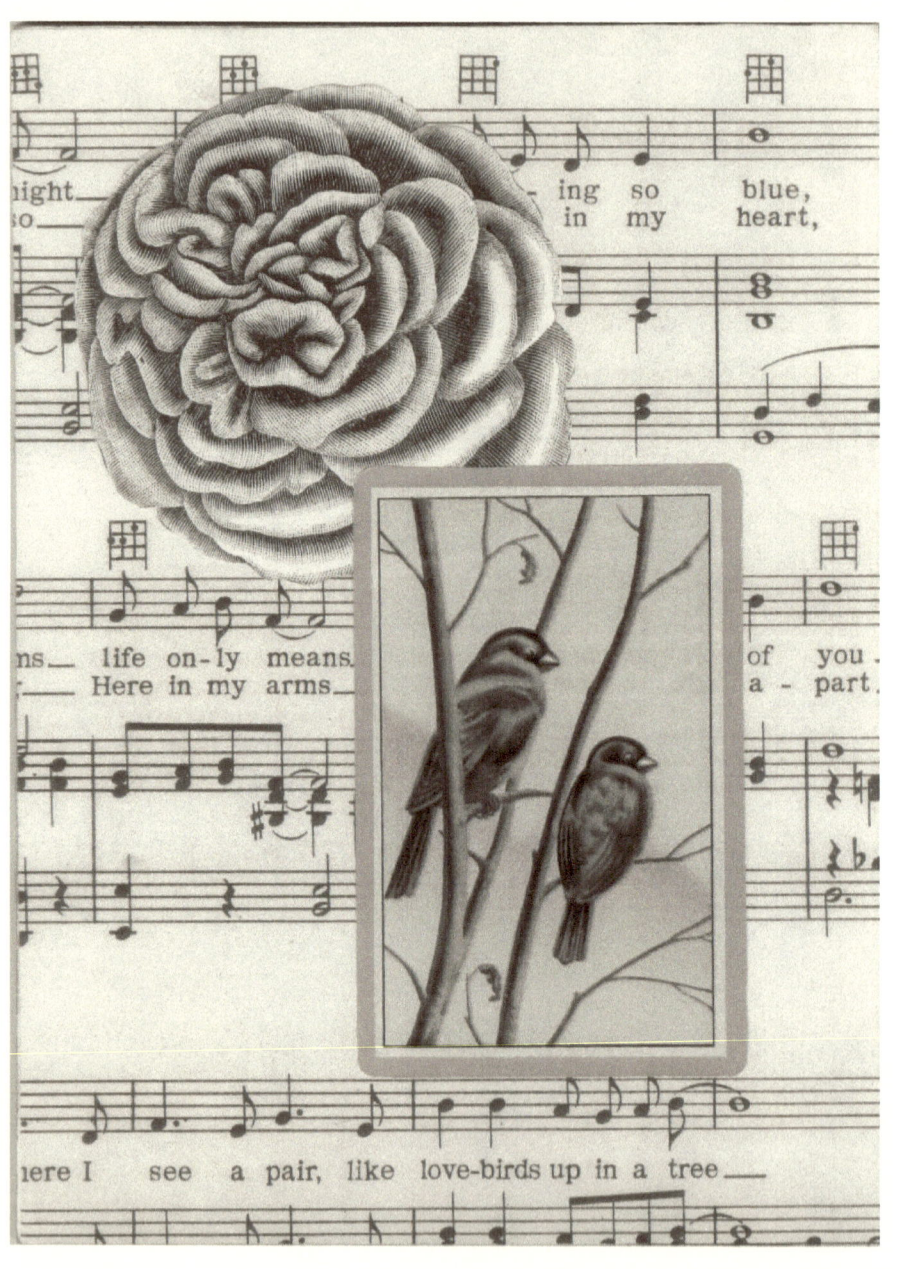

Chapter Six

Embracing the Insignificant

> I like trees because they seem more resigned to the
> way they have to live than other things do.
> —*Willa Cather*

Most cancer patients will attest to the debilitating effects of chemotherapy. Fatigue, hair loss, nausea, and general malaise accompany the treatment.

However, appreciation of your surroundings does not have to diminish. Certainly, a chemically induced slowdown will interfere with your ability to involve yourself physically with your environment. However, higher-level thinking can establish new and rewarding connections with your surroundings. (The concept of higher-level thinking will be discussed in detail in chapter 10.)

From an easy chair or lounger placed near a window, or a beach chair on a front porch, you can observe, contemplate, and mentally digest a wide variety of situations:

- The sun rising at dawn and setting in the evening
- Traffic, children, and workers creating the sounds of life
- The branches of trees and the patterns of flowers responding to nature's design
- The falling of snow and the patter of raindrops as they refresh the earth
- Vendors plying their trade to children and adults
- Street games being played by children who prefer a non-park environment
- Rediscover radio: A small battery-powered AM/FM radio can be an invaluable companion, especially on days when fatigue or nausea dominates. I discovered NPR—National Public Radio—

and find it a spirited listening experience. Likewise, music and sports may accomplish the same task.

The changing seasons present a panorama for "embracing the insignificant." Colors that were taken for granted, changes in temperature that were accepted without notice, changing cloud formations, and shortened days become a feast for the eyes and the senses.

I believe that sustenance can be absorbed from your surroundings. Depression and fatigue thrive on loneliness and isolation. The simple plan outlined above can bring the outside world into a body that is repelling against it.

END QUOTES

Spring, thy name is color.

—Libbie Fudim

The sky is the daily bread of the eyes.

—Ralph Waldo Emerson

Speak to the earth, and it shall teach thee.

—The Bible

Autumn carries more gold in its hand than all the other seasons.

—Jim Bishop

When elephants fight, it is the grass that suffers.

—African proverb

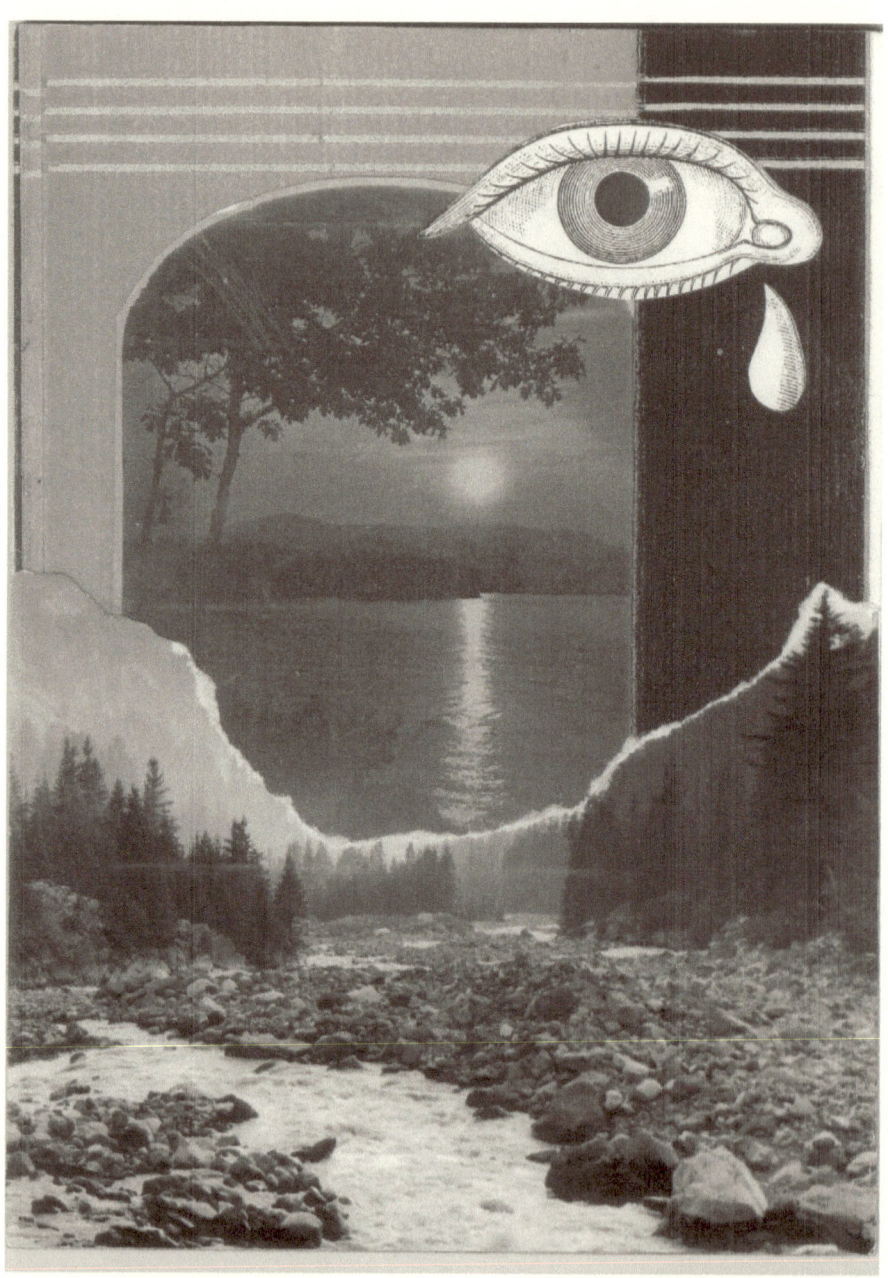

Chapter Seven

Moving beyond Grief

Nobody can give you wiser advice than yourself.

—*Cicero*

The grief of victimization is a powerful agent. Mourning for what had been and envying the past propels the mind into internal turmoil. And there it festers until your "mourning period" becomes a way of life.

Grief can be the quicksand of cancer—pulling you down into an abyss of depression. Although medications can be prescribed to fight depression, I suggest you seek solutions by redefining your attitude toward life.

Positive expectancy is a worthwhile bridge to attitude adjustment. Your vision of a brighter tomorrow, a sunnier future, and satisfactory results on PET/CAT scans will buoy your spirits and help the movement beyond grief.

Take steps to ensure that the mood of the moment does not become a permanent state of grief. Moods reflect temporary situations. The bubble of grief surrounding you can be ruptured through determination. Ask yourself:

- *Is my grief a form of self-pity designed as penitence for creating this situation?*
- *Am I mourning for happy times prior to illness?*
- *Is my grief a method of control over a highly volatile illness?*
- *Am I compensating for my loss of dignity and self-respect by creating an aura of despair?*

If your answers favor a *yes,* then perhaps you should consider the idea that you are fostering a deleterious effect on your body. Misery and mourning are nonproductive activities.

Start to create an environment that builds better mental health. Approach the goal in little steps. Establish a vision of normalcy. Rather than justifying your mourning, redefine your life's direction.

Enjoying rewards, new garments, different foods, visits to new places, or meeting friends for lunch may serve as an impetus to attitude readjustment.

Figuratively speaking, "The mind is its own place, and in itself can make a heaven of hell and a hell of heaven."

END QUOTES

Laugh and the world laughs with you; Weep, and you cry alone.

—Ella W. Wilcox

Hope springs eternal in the human breast; Man never is, but always to be blest.

—Alexander Pope

Acceptance is not submission; it is acknowledgement of the facts of the situation. Then deciding what you're going to do about it.

—Kathleen Casey Thiesen

One cannot get through life without pain ... What we can do is choose how to use the pain life presents to us.

—Dr. Bernie Siegel

There are two ways of meeting difficulties: you alter the difficulties or you alter yourself to meet them.

—Phyllis Bottome

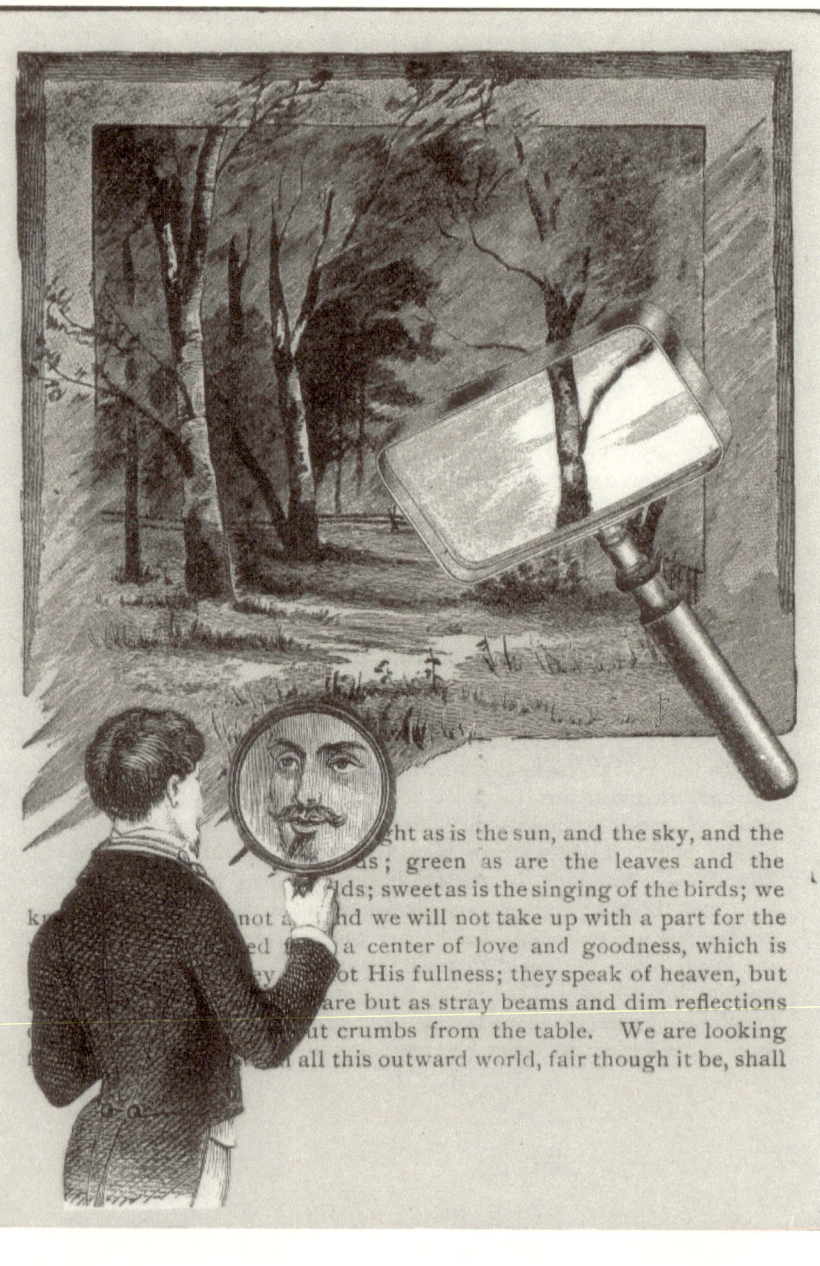

ght as is the sun, and the sky, and the
s; green as are the leaves and the
lds; sweet as is the singing of the birds; we
k not a d we will not take up with a part for the
d a center of love and goodness, which is
ot His fullness; they speak of heaven, but
are but as stray beams and dim reflections
t crumbs from the table. We are looking
all this outward world, fair though it be, shall

Chapter Eight

Searching for the Truth

The presence of those seeking the truth is infinitely to
be preferred to those who think they've found it.

—*Terry Pratchett*

Is cancer a truth-altering disease? On the other hand, has your illness given
you the insight to decipher the truth? Let us define what is meant by "the
truth."

Searching for the truth is looking for *absolutes*. An "absolute" smacks
of finality—an unswerving decision of acceptance. No discussion, no moot
points, no flip-flopping. Absolute truths are present in religion, science,
philosophy, politics, and mathematics.

Fellow patients, I do not ask you to abandon your acceptance of absolute
faith in what you believe. What I do ask is that you use your higher-level
thinking skills to evaluate the foundation of your absolutism.

Religious Truth

For some people, a diagnosis of cancer has a "faith weakening" effect. For
others, it may bring them closer to their belief in a higher deity.

The Bible has the potential for becoming your source of sustenance.
Specific passages and recollections may provide you, the reader, with the
strength needed to combat your insidious disease. For many patients, hope
and faith are inextricably combined to help them see through the fog of their
disease. Faith can provide the courage to face life.

Faith looks forward, while grief looks backward. Bemoaning your
unfortunate "inheritance" is not a medicinally positive attitude. What has
happened has happened. Let it go. Playing the blame game is nonproductive
and enervating.

Just as renewal is present in the trees of winter and the tundras of the far North, your faith can nourish your fight for life.

Let us now address those who question the existence of a higher being, or Creator. Can hope exist without faith in a supreme being?

We have here a question of opinion versus conviction. Many people share the opinion that the Bible has undergone stages of translation from archaic languages, myriad changes by scribes to reflect conditions in the societies of that era, and inaccurate interpretations of original text.

For many people, the Bible is good literature but not the law of the land. It may serve as a "manual" for behavior, but not as the words of the Creator.

Differences may also exist in fixed notions of a hereafter. Some of the faithful may see heaven not as a place, but rather as a state of mind.

Others may regard heaven as the seeking of perfection. Beyond that, some see "termination" as an ultimate power failure: a cessation of all physical and mental systems, a power plant shut down. With these choices in mind, you may ask:

- *Is there a best way to die?*
- *If my illness is my Creator's will, why take medication and undergo procedures to stay alive?*
- *Would I consider facing death as life's greatest challenge?*

These are challenging questions requiring substantial thought. Perhaps cancer is a "truth-altering disease," enabling its victims to construct answers. Do these answers appear as blinding sources of inspiration? Or perhaps they appear as a form of introspection—a pacifying admittance of inner beliefs.

END QUOTES

The truth is rarely pure, and never simple.

—Oscar Wilde

*'Tis strange—but true; for truth is always strange; Stranger
than fiction.*

—Lord Byron

Let us all work together to stop "truth decay."

—Unknown

Truth is so precarious some people use it sparingly.

—Unknown

*Few people seek to discover truth; most of us seek to confirm
our errors and perpetuate our prejudices.*

—Unknown

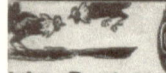
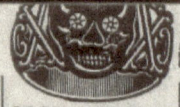
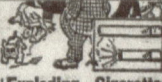
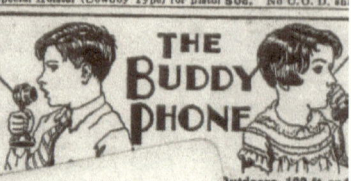
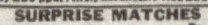
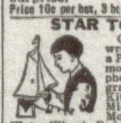
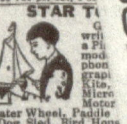
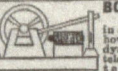
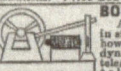
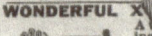
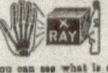
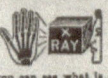
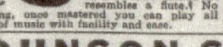
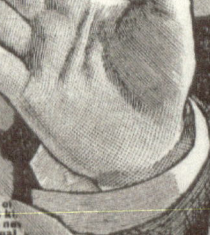
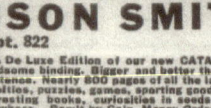

Chapter Nine

Funny Bones

It takes more facial muscles to frown than to smile.
—*Medical fact*

Cancer patients become inured to the countless blood tests, probes, treatments, and procedures that undoubtedly work to obliterate a sense of humor. We overlook the salubrious effects of laughter.

How, then, can patients retain an optimistic, positive, and rosy attitude with dark clouds hovering over the horizon? Simply stated, how can we retain our sense of humor?

Not an easy answer. However, your sense of humor, although diminished, can be rekindled. The step between pessimism and optimism is realism. Realism enables the cancer patient to accept the present and live for the day. Humor then becomes part of the daily routine. Recover what you may have lost.

Presented here are six humorous challenges for higher-level thinking exercises. See how well you can do. Naturally, the unaffected are expected to attain a perfect score—or is the bar being set too high?

1. Two Roman citizens are traveling along an ancient highway. They see this sign:

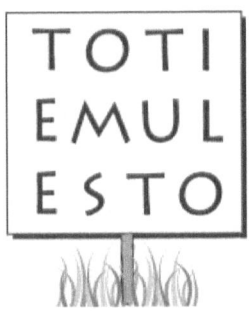

What is the English translation?

2. Mr. A's peacock wanders into Mr. B's backyard and lays an egg. Who owns the egg—Mr. A or Mr. B?
3. Which is correct: "Lemons *is* sweet" or "Lemons *are* sweet"?
4. Why do we park on a driveway but drive on a parkway?
5. Why do we put garments in a suitcase and suits in a garment bag?
6. Why do we put cargo in a ship but a shipment in a car?

Answers:

1. To tie mules to.
2. No problem. Peacocks are males and cannot lay eggs. Peahens lay eggs.
3. Neither. Lemons are *sour.*
4–6. Because English can be a very confusing language.

Have you wondered why your elbow is called a "funny bone"? In layman's terms, the large bone of the upper arm is the "humerus"—closely allied to the word *humorous,* or funny.

END QUOTES

He who laughs, lasts.

—Unknown

You don't stop laughing because you grow old; you grow old because you stop laughing.

—Michael Pritchard

Laughter is the sun that drives winter from the human face.

—Victor Hugo

Laughter is a medicine with no side effects.

—Unknown

Laughter can be heard farther than weeping.

—Unknown

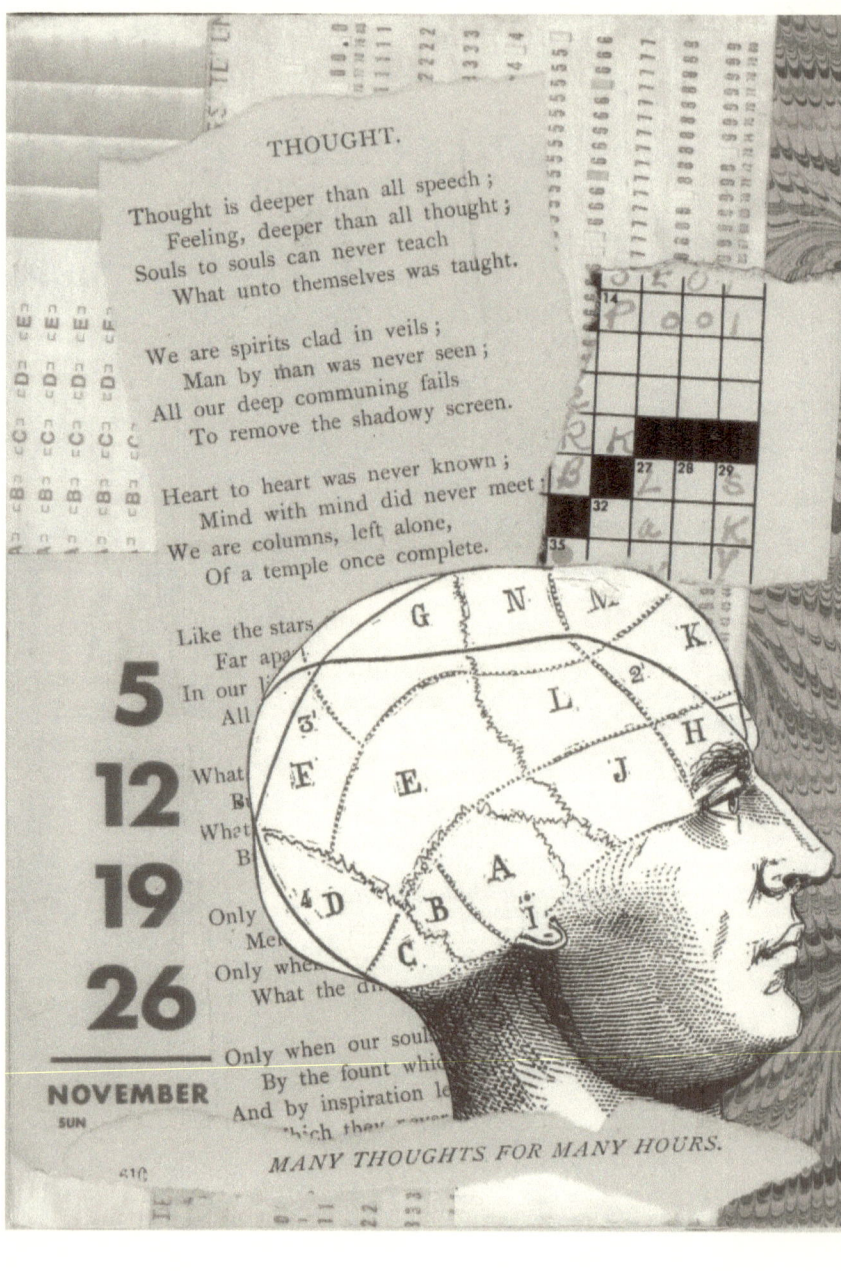

THOUGHT.

Thought is deeper than all speech;
Feeling, deeper than all thought;
Souls to souls can never teach
What unto themselves was taught.

We are spirits clad in veils;
Man by man was never seen;
All our deep communing fails
To remove the shadowy screen.

Heart to heart was never known;
Mind with mind did never meet;
We are columns, left alone,
Of a temple once complete.

Like the stars
Far apa
In our l
All

What
B
What
B

Only
Me
Only whe
What the d

Only when our soul
By the fount which
And by inspiration le
hich they

5

12

19

26

NOVEMBER
SUN

MANY THOUGHTS FOR MANY HOURS.

Chapter Ten

Higher-Level Thinking

I think, therefore I am.

—*Rene Descartes*

In this chapter, we will explore the cancer patient's relationship to the process of thinking. Questions will be posed to focus on chemotherapy and its effects on lucidity, memory, and the ability to process information. In addition, attention will be directed to concentration, confusion, and inattention.

Please consider the following rhetorical questions:

- *Can chemotherapy and/or related cancer treatments affect the thinking processes?*
- *Are friends and loved ones doing you a favor when they do your thinking for you?*
- *If an erosion of brain cells does occur, what can be done to counter that condition?*
- *How would you define "thinking?"*
- *Does fatigue and/or pain set limits on the thinking process?*

These questions will be addressed in the content of this chapter.

Cancer should not eliminate or diminish the thinking process. Certainly, fatigue and/or pain may affect the intensity and duration of analyzing, reasoning, and contemplation. Questioning and probing cancer-related issues are still very much in use. Perhaps mental gymnastics will not be as popular as before, but this cannot be ruled out. If you view your illness as a "covenant of death," it will start to shut down your creative juices.

To encourage your thinking processes, avoid having others think for you. Although well meaning, this favor is counterproductive. Select your own clothing for the day; make your own breakfast, lunch, or dinner choices; and be part of family decisions.

41

Related directly to your illness:

- Keep a listing of all medicines used for chemotherapy, fusions, and injections.
- Maintain a calendar of appointments for medical issues.
- Participate in all decisions concerning your treatment.
- Maintain a file of literature—using folders—about your particular type of cancer.
- Obtain results from CAT and PET scans and blood tests and develop a filing system.
- Know the names, titles, and functions of your medical office staff, including physicians.
- There are many nonmedical activities that cancer patients can use to exercise their thinking skills:
- The daily newspaper usually prints a crossword puzzle waiting to be completed.
- Keeping a diary provides a daily activity.
- Create a family tree.
- Start a blog on your computer.
- Write a poem.

THE ART OF SELF-QUESTIONING

Self-questioning will arouse your curiosity, revitalize your thinking, and encourage silent contemplation. You have earned the right to question. Of prime concern is the answer to this question: "Why me?"

Answer: "Why *not* me?"

Was a contract violated? Was there a commitment from anyone that, at age seventy-five, I would be faced with the most serious challenge of my life?

Questions that you pose do not have to be complex. You may wish to think about questions that review religious beliefs, fatalistic theories, and political or social issues.

My questions come to me at all times of the day and night. However, they appear clearer and deeper during twilight sleep or upon awakening in the predawn hours. Perhaps the mind is freer at that time, refreshed from a few hours of sleep. A pad is kept on my night table and used to record these thoughts before they are lost to the "dawn's early light."

THE ART OF QUESTIONING

In the play *Cyrano De Bergerac*, by Edmond Rostand, the art of questioning reaches extraordinary heights. Note that answers are not forthcoming, but the questions from Cyrano come at a rapid pace.

Cyrano is a brave soldier in the palace guard of the king of France. He is a gifted poet and an expert swordsman. However, there is something very unusual about Cyrano. An enormous nose handicaps him, causing great sensitivity to that part of his face. It is believed that Cyrano has killed several men who dared to give him strange looks or make comments about his nose.

CYRANO DE BERGERAC
By Edmond Rostand

CYRANO: Tell me why you're looking at my nose.

THE MEDDLER (*petrified*): I ...

CYRANO (*moving toward him*): Do you find it surprising?

THE MEDDLER (*stepping back*): You're mistaken, my lord ...

CYRANO: Is it limp and dangling, like an elephant's trunk?

THE MEDDLER (*stepping back again*): I didn't ...

CYRANO: Or hooked like an owl's beak?

THE MEDDLER: I ...
CYRANO: Does its color seem unhealthy to you?

THE MEDDLER: Sir!
CYRANO: Is its shape obscene?

THE MEDDLER: Not at all!

CYRANO: Then why that disdainful expression? Do you find it, perhaps, a little too large?

THE MEDDLER (*stammering*): Oh, no, it's quite small ... very small ... diminutive ...

CYRANO: What! How dare you accuse me of anything so ridiculous? A small nose? *My* nose? You've gone too far!

THE MEDDLER: Please, sir, I ...
THE MEDDLER: I ...

CYRANO: Or a fly walking on it? What's unusual about it?

THE MEDDLER: Nothing, I ...

CYRANO: Is it a startling sight?

THE MEDDLER: Sir, I've been careful not to look at it!

CYRANO: Would you please tell me why?

THE MEDDLER: I was ...
THE MEDDLER: Please, sir, I ...

CYRANO: My nose is *enormous*, you snub-nosed, flat-faced wretch! I carry it with pride, because a big nose is a sign of affability, kindness, courtesy, wit, generosity, and courage. I have all those qualities, but you can never hope to have any of them, since the ignoble face that my hand is about to meet above your collar ... (*slaps him and THE MEDDLER cries out in pain*) ... has no more glory, nobility, poetry, quaintness, vivacity, or grandeur—no more *nose*, in short—than the face that my boot ... (*turns him around by the shoulders*) ... is about to meet below your waist! (*kicks him*)

VALVERT: Just watch his face when he hears what I have to say to him! (*walks up to CYRANO, who observes him and stands in front of him with a fatuous expression*) You have a nose that ... Your nose is ... um ... very big.

CYRANO (*gravely*): Yes, very.

VALVERT (*laughing*): Ha!

CYRANO (*with perfect calm*): Is that all?

VALVERT: Well ...

CYRANO: I'm afraid your speech was a little short, young man. You could have said ... oh, all sorts of things, varying your tone to fit your words. Let me give you a few examples.

- **In an aggressive tone:** "If I had a nose like that, I'd have it amputated!"

- **Friendly:** "The end of it must get wet when you drink from a cup. Why don't you use a bowl?"

- **Curious:** "What do you use that long container for? Do you keep your pens and scissors in it?"

- **Gracious:** "What a kind man you are! You love birds so much that you've given them a perch to roost on."

- **Truculent:** "When you light your pipe and the smoke comes out of your nose, the neighbors must think a chimney has caught fire!"

- **Solicitous:** "Be careful when you walk: with all that weight on your head, you could easily lose your balance and fall."

- **Thoughtful:** "You ought to put an awning over it, to keep its color from fading in the sun."

- **Flippant:** "That tusk must be convenient to hang your hat on."

- **Grandiloquent:** "No wind but the mighty Arctic blast, majestic nose, could ever give you a cold from one end to the other!"

- **Dramatic:** "When it bleeds, it must be like the Red Sea!"

- **Admiring:** "What a sign for a perfume shop!"

- **Lyrical:** "Is that a seashell, and are you Triton risen from the sea?"

- **Naive:** "Is that monument open to the public?"

- **Respectful:** "One look at your face, sir, is enough to tell me you are indeed a man of substance."

- **Rustic:** "That don't look like a nose to me. It's either a big cucumber or a little watermelon."

- **Military:** "The enemy is charging! Aim your cannon!"

- **Practical:** "A nose like that has one advantage: it keeps your feet dry in the rain."

There, now you have an inkling of what you might have said to me if you were witty and a man of letters. Unfortunately, you're totally witless and a man of very few letters: only the four that spell the word, "fool." But even if you had the intelligence to invent remarks like those I've given you as examples, you would not have been able to entertain me with them. You would have spoken no more than half the first syllable of the first word, because such jesting is a privilege that I grant only to myself.

Have you counted the number of questions posed by Cyrano? You may be surprised.

AUDIOBOOKS

Many fiction and nonfiction books have been recorded. This is a wonderful way for people who are too fatigued to read to keep up with the latest literature.

This chapter focused on strategies to stimulate thinking. Remember that you control your ability to keep brain cells alive with activities that encourage mind power.

END QUOTES

*Good thoughts bear good fruit, bad thoughts bear bad fruit—
and man is his own gardener.*

—James Allen

*Thinking is the hardest work there is, which is probably the
reason so few engage in it.*

—Henry Ford

*To think too long about doing something often becomes its
undoing.*

—Eva Young

*Some people get lost in thought because it's such unfamiliar
territory.*

—G. Behn

Think wrongly, if you please, but in all cases think for yourself.
—Doris Lessing

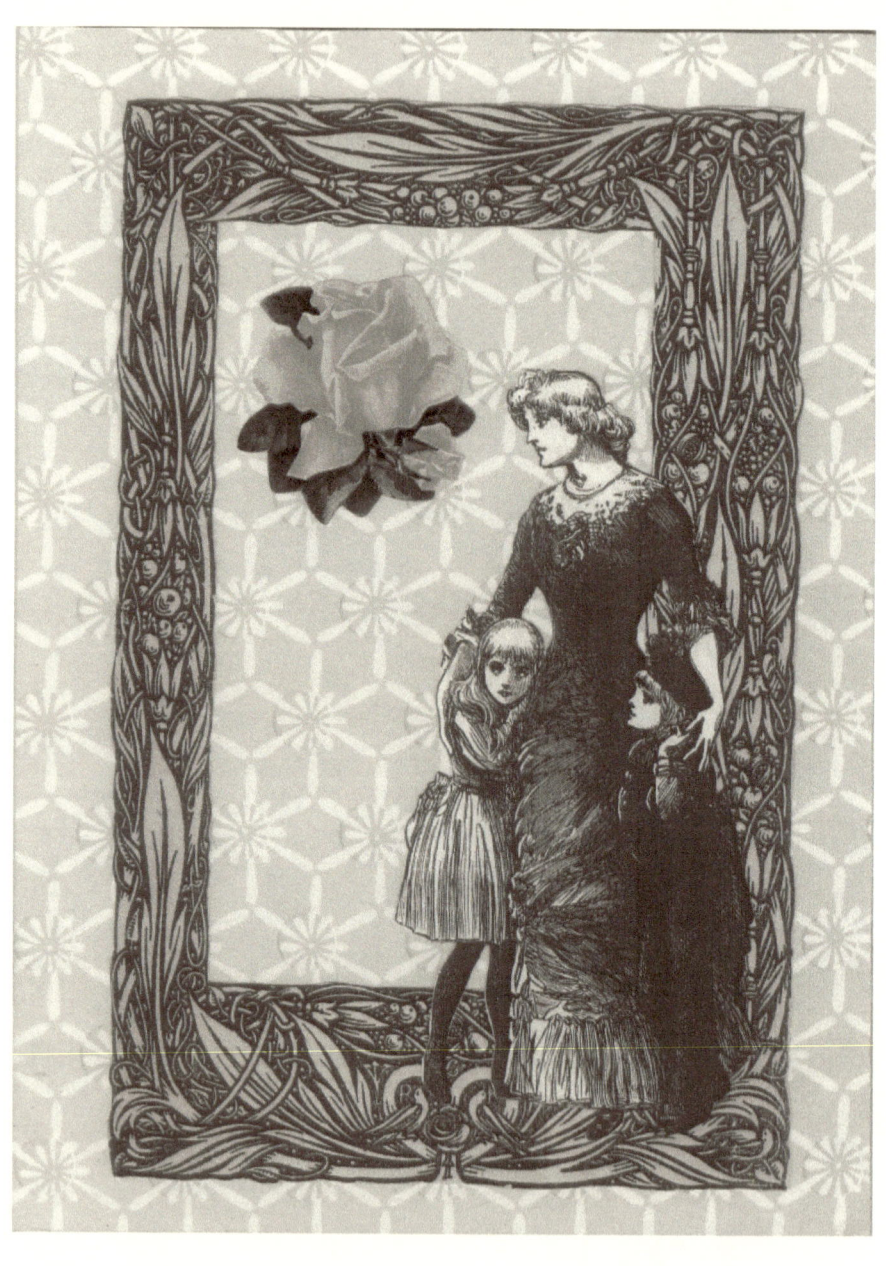

Chapter Eleven

Mothers with Cancer

All mothers are physically handicapped. They have
only two hands.

—Unknown

All cancer patients encounter challenges. However, mothers with cancer have an inordinate amount of demands. These demands cannot be overlooked. They are disruptive, complicated, and anxiety laden. This chapter attempts to analyze, discuss, and treat the problems presented to mothers of babies, toddlers, and preschool children.

Cancer is a disease of inconvenience. Physically it ravages the body, socially it strains relationships with spouses and friends, and financially it is an economic burden.

For mothers in particular, it is particularly disruptive. Medical appointments, chemotherapy schedules, and frequent blood and diagnostic tests create havoc with children's feeding, sleep, and play date schedules.

TODDLERS

Ideally, daily assistance from friends, relatives, or per-hour helpers can be comforting. Realistically, this help may not be forthcoming for many mothers. Local clergy may be in a position to enlist volunteers as "home assistants." Likewise, cancer care organizations may provide help in this area.

Care must be exercised in the prevention of pill ingestion by toddlers who confuse candy-colored pills for a candy treat. Take steps to secure your pills in safe havens far out of reach of curious little hands.

Mothers taking chemotherapy are prone to reduced white blood cells—an important ingredient for fighting infection. A diminished immune system "red flags" the changing of diapers and training pants. As a precautionary routine, avoid direct contact with fecal matter. Seek assistance in this area. If not possible, wash hands carefully and frequently.

DAY CARE

Nursery and preschool programs offer a welcome respite for mothers. If financially possible, and realistic for transporting back and forth, day care is ideal. Naturally, medical treatments must coincide with the day care schedule.

TALKING WITH CHILDREN

Whether or not to tell children about mother's illness appears to be a three-phase procedure.

> **Phase One:** No fault. Mothers know their children well. Be alert to youngsters who may be blaming themselves for their mother's illness. Assure the children that in no way could anything they have done, or said, had any effect on their mother's condition.

> **Phase Two:** Contagion. Children may harbor the fear of "catching" the illness. Shying away from a mother's hugs and kisses may be a warning sign. Once again, assure them that the sickness cannot be caught from another person.

> **Phase Three:** Age ready. Mothers should monitor their children's reaction to the process of communicating. Scaling your explanation up or down according to the age level is highly recommended. The choice of words, concern over the "fear factor," and maintaining normalcy are all worthy of consideration.

HOUSEHOLD CHORES

Fatigue, appointments, and tests may hamper the degree to which household chores are accomplished. Do not confuse the present with the past—what was, was! Adopt laborsaving strategies to work smarter. I have outlined several:

Meals: Increase reliance on the microwave, leftovers, frozen foods, and contributions from relatives and friends. Baby formula and complete lines of baby foods are readily available. Perhaps bulk buying, if possible, can stock the pantry with an adequate supply.

To diminish dishwashing chores—whether by hand or machine—utilize paper or plastic plates and utensils with increased frequency.

Spousal Assistance: Erratic nighttime sleep schedules, predawn feedings, and bouts of crying may tax the limits of a mother's strength. Utilizing spousal assistance is imperative. If not forthcoming, the help of relatives and clergy to discuss with the spouse the need for greater assistance may be necessary.

Home Cleanliness: Housekeeping chores to maintain a degree of hygiene in the home are essential. No doubt that scrubbing, mopping, and scouring require an inordinate amount of energy. If household help is not available, mothers should adjust their cleaning to activities within reason.

When living quarters become messy and grubby, tensions increase and depression takes hold. The eyes perceive a shabby environment, and the brain compares the situation to pre-cancer times.

Scale down the degree of spotlessness, but do not let the situation deteriorate to the extent of slovenliness. Laundering, sweeping, and vacuuming schedules should be adjusted but not eliminated.

Shopping: The modern supermarket is immense. Its size can present an issue to mothers who have difficulty walking. To assist mothers with the chore of walking, utilize the shopping cart. It is an invaluable asset as a "walker," as well as a carriage for children. Mothers are urged to clip their pocketbooks to the safety strap as a security measure.

Handicapped spaces are closer to entrances and limit the amount of walking. Naturally, a handicap placard must be displayed within the car. These permits are available at your doctor's request.

To conserve strength while shopping, prepare a grocery list prior to departure. If possible, enlist the help of a concerned neighbor who must do his or her marketing at the same time.

Another alternative is to consider buying groceries online and having them delivered.

PERSONAL APPEARANCE

"Looking good, feeling better," is the motto of an organization devoted to maintaining a level of acceptable appearance by female cancer patients.

Hair loss may require a wig or a hairpiece that complements your face. Makeup may be required to replace eyebrows or eyelashes that have been lost due to chemo. The hairpiece or turban selected will do much to enhance mental attitude as well as appearance.

CLOTHING

If weight loss has occurred to a significant degree, a visit to a local shop may be in order. To accompany a new set of duds, mothers may wish to splurge on a manicure or pedicure as an elevating step.

SINGLE MOTHERS

In addition to all the issues discussed in this chapter, single mothers with cancer have concerns of vital importance.

With no spousal assistance, the burden of providing round-the-clock care for babies and toddlers is significant. If economically feasible, live-in help or assistance from relatives would help greatly.

Many single mothers with cancer may still be working on a full- or part-time basis. Employer-generated stress puts additional strains on this serious situation. Schedules must be adjusted to fit the work schedule.

Decisions that single mothers may consider involve school and PTA activities. The degree to which a single mother with cancer can participate in after-school or evening activities is a choice that should be carefully considered.

SCHOOL ACTIVITIES

At the middle and high school level, parental involvement with sports and academic activities may be time consuming. Spousal reliance on sharing evening meetings or attending sports events may relieve a mother of some responsibility.

Mothers should also consider informing the school about their illness. This is a decision that only the patient can make.

As a father and grandfather, I cannot presume to understand fully the crucial issues facing mothers with cancer. Their fortitude is admirable, and their level of frustration must be major.

An adage says, "Walk a mile in my shoes."

Dear mothers, I wish I could, but the closest I can come to that is looking into your hearts.

END QUOTES

Children are the anchors that hold a mother to life.

—Sophocles

There is no such thing as a nonworking mother.

—Hester Mundis

The joys of motherhood are never fully experienced until all the children are in bed.

—Unknown

When you are a mother, you are never really alone in your thoughts. A mother always has to think twice, once for herself and once for her child.

—Sophia Loren

The hand that rocks the cradle is the hand that rules the world.

—William Ross Wallace

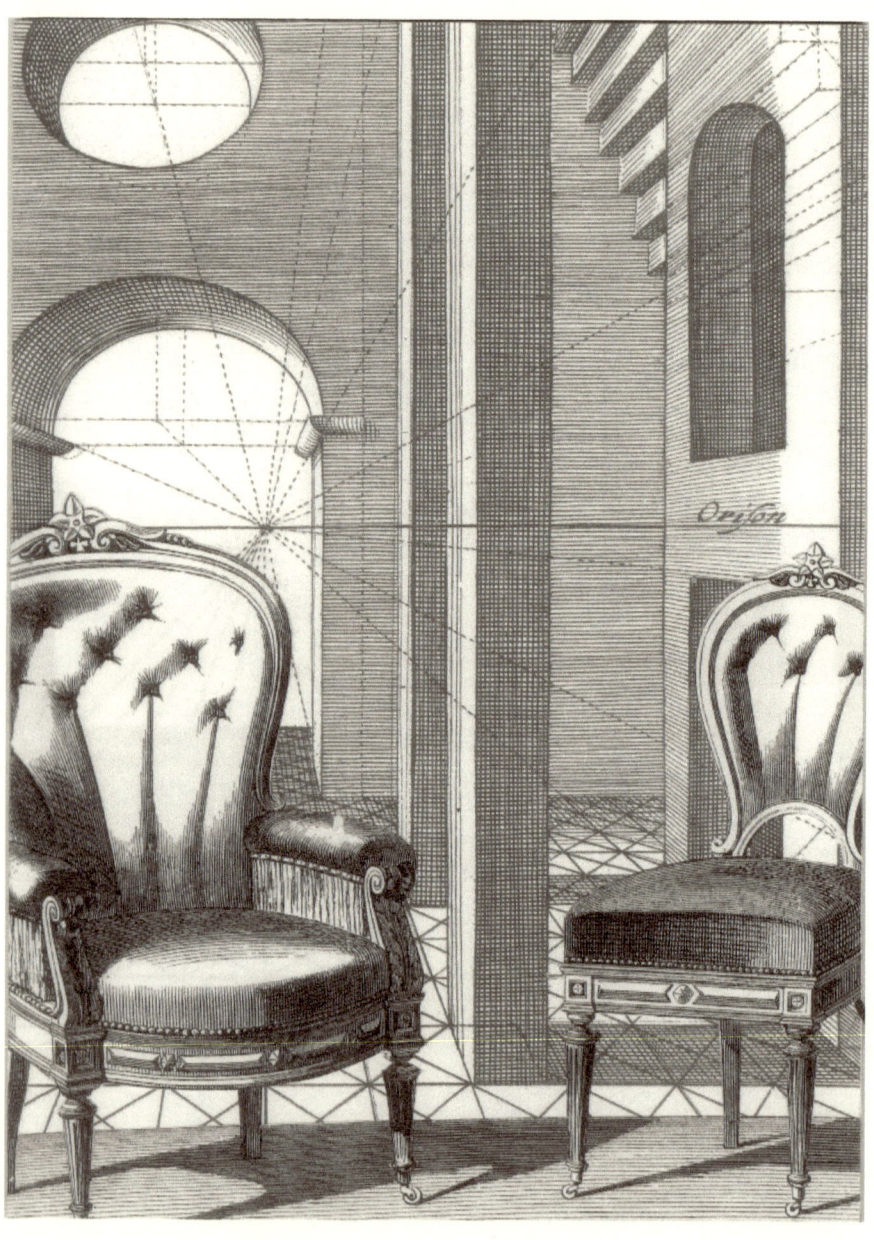

Chapter Twelve

Creating Comfort Zones

Summer afternoon; to me those have always been the
two most beautiful words in the English language.
—*Henry James*

In the first two lines of Samuel Taylor Coleridge's poem about the Emperor
Kubla Khan, we learn that he has ordered the construction of a palace of
opulent comfort:

In Xanadu did Kubla Khan
A stately pleasure dome decree.

Creating comfort zones, or areas of quiet pleasure, will be a valuable asset
to bolstering your immune system.

How, then, can comfort zones be created? Simply, there are areas in and
around your home conducive to contentment. A favorite chair, a folding
beach chair, or a lounger, moved outside, may radiate cheer.

Considering seasonal adjustments, I have become accustomed to sitting
in my driveway on a folding chair, gladdened by the sight of neighborhood
people.

The sights and sounds around me brighten my day. Connections are
made through visual and auditory stimuli. In inclement weather, I moved
my comfort zone into my garage—with the door wide open. I could feast
my eyes on the environment.

Derive pleasure from your comfort zone. There are times when I resemble
a fisherman—hoping to catch a neighbor, a repairperson, or the postman,
someone who will stop for a moment for a friendly chat. My cell phone often
accompanies me on these outside jaunts.

Am I stopping to smell the roses? Probably. Self-contentedness exists in many ways. Not grandiose, but satisfying—quiet pleasure from quiet sources.

Blue skies, cloud formations, and swaying trees are part of my comfort zone. Emergency vehicles with sirens blasting may intrude upon my satisfying outdoor rest. However, a comfortable return is imminent.

In your comfort zone, you accept what you are—not what you want to be. Children build tree houses, adolescents have club rooms, and college students share frat houses. All comfort zones. All provide contentment and assurance.

Enjoy your restrictive hiatus. Letter writing, listening to the radio, or just observing the rest of the world going by are part and parcel of your comfort zone.

The amount of time spent by yourself depends on several considerations. Mealtimes, bathroom breaks, weather changes, and fatigue may abbreviate your zone time. This will even out over an extended period.

Comfort is where you find it. Explore and discover your "tree house."

It's great to be a kid again!

END QUOTES

Change is what people fear most.

—Fyodor Dostoyevsky

The key to change ... is to let go of fear.

—Rosanne Cash

I am happy and content because I think I am.

—Alain-Rene Lesage

I finally figured out the only reason to be alive is to enjoy it.

—Rita Mae Brown

The best place to find a helping hand is at the end of your own arm.

—Swedish proverb

ng parts, and so
are uncoördinated
benign or malign,
they encroach upon
like "cancers."

CHAPTER IX.—*Continued*   to which m

	PAGE
IV. Disturbances That Work In	181
1. Internal Disturbances	181
(a) Formative Disturbances advancing	181
(b) Mechanical Interferences Tumors	182
(c) Responsive Maladjustments ar state,	183
(d) Hereditary Handicaps	183
2. External Disturbances case	184
(a) Thermal Factors	4
(b) Chemical Factors	4
(c) Barometric Factors	84
(d) Mechanical Factors	
(e) Biological Factors	
V. Sources of Pathological Knowledge	
VI. The Control of Disease	

vo cab u lar y (vŏ kab′ū ler′i
words used by a people, class,
will increase your vocabulary.
with their meanings. *n.*, p

of

can cer (kan′sər)   a very harmful growth
in the body. Cancer tends to spread and
destroy the healthy tissues and organs

Surgery and radiation are the

tissues and organs

nature of cancer
symptoms have

Microscopic	203
3. Embryonic	207
IV. Comparati	207
chances of successful treatment.	207
2. Tunicates	209
3. Amphi	

199
199

Chapter Thirteen

The Vocabulary of Cancer

Words are seductive and dangerous material and
should be used with caution.

—*Unknown*

Cancer patients face the challenge of learning a new language. Not some foreign tongue spoken in a far-off land or on a remote island. This new language is the "language of pathology"—a cryptic and mystical medical language that interprets test results. Unknown to the layman, but familiar to the oncologist, these polysyllabic words defy the patient.

Written without contempt or insolence, the language defies the layman's knowledge and demands interpretation from knowledgeable sources.

I recall reading this sentence from one of my medical reports: "Multimodular conglomerated malignant lung mass in the right upper lung extending to the right hilum along with multiple bilateral hilar, subcarinal and right paratracheal metastatic lymphadenopathy."

This tongue twister and mind twister cries out for interpretation.

Should medical reports resemble mystery stories? They are not mysterious for physicians, only the patients who are directly affected by the information.

In her poem "Pretty Words," Elinor Wylie classifies her words: pretty words, smooth words, tender words, bright words, lazy words, and cool words.

It appears that the various types of cancers produce their own vocabulary. These words will appear in all reports about your diagnosis, treatment, and prognosis. The layman searches each report for familiar words that offer a glimmer of hope and indications of improvement.

We look for "comfortable" words with hints of recovery. Sometimes they are difficult to find. But look we must because hope springs eternal.

As a result of PET (positron-emission tomography) and CAT (computerized axial tomography) scans, pathology reports alter their language to conform to the particular cancer: bladder, bone, breast, cervical, colorectal, esophageal, gastrointestinal, head and neck, Hodgkin's, kidney, larynx, leukemia, lung, lymphoma, melanoma, myeloma, oral, ovarian, prostate, sarcoma, skin, testicular, and thyroid.

Each area mentioned produces its own vocabulary. It is overwhelming to consider the number of polysyllabic words used to describe the twenty-five areas mentioned above. These "jawbreakers" reveal pertinent information needed to establish protocols of treatment.

Try your best to familiarize yourself with these words. Friends and relatives who read your reports may request an explanation—a breaking of *The DaVinci Code* of cancer.

ABBREVIATIONS

Laboratory blood tests present another challenge: the dreaded abbreviation. Blood tests in particular use a system of shorthand to categorize blood components: NEU, LYM, MON, EOS, BAS, RBC, HGB, HCT, MCV, MCH, RDW, PLT.

Your phlebotomist or oncologist can offer a brief explanation of each abbreviation. Disclosure of each one will make your blood tests more meaningful.

Words can be music to our ears or objects of torment. Words can be stressful or calming. The choice is up to you.

END QUOTES

Words can destroy. What we call each other ultimately becomes what we think of each other, and it matters.

—Jeanne J. Kirkpatrick

Everyone hears only what he understands.

—Goethe

Words hang like wash on the line, blowing in the winds of the mind.

—Ram Das

Words sometimes serve as a smoke screen to obscure truth, rather than as a searchlight to reveal it.

—Unknown

SMILE is the longest word in the world. There's a "mile" between the first and last letters in the word.

—English pun

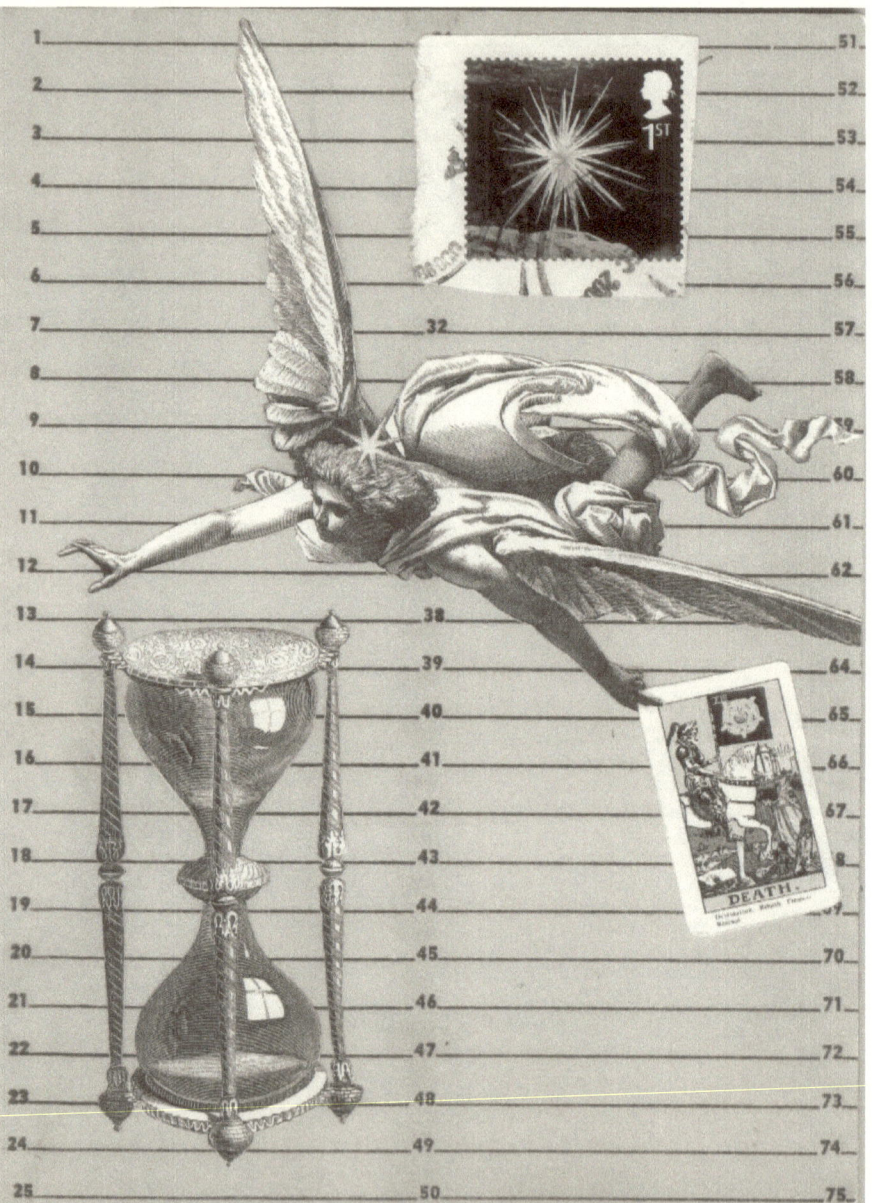

Chapter Fourteen

Death Re-viewed

Death is a delightful hiding place for weary people.
—Herodotus

Dear colleague in illness, you deserve to know why, in a book that purports to be inspirational and hopeful, a section on death has been included.

The decision was not an easy one. However, statistically, realistically, and mystically, the decision became apparent. Death can be inspirational, and as you will soon see in the following context, can be re-viewed from an unusual perspective.

Not all famous allusions to death have been ominous and foreboding. A collection of elevating and, I might say, humorous quotations have been included for your consideration.

But first let us return to the factors that make this section inclusive:

1. **Statistically** I recently called the resource research unit of the American Cancer Society to solicit answers to several questions relevant to cancer deaths in the United States.

> **Question:** "How many people are expected to die from cancer in 2007?"
> **Answer:** "559,000."
> **Question:** "How many people die each day from cancer-related illness?"
> **Answer:** "1,500."
> **Question:** "Is cancer the number one cause of death in the United States?"
> **Answer:** "No. Heart-related deaths are first. Cancer-related deaths are second. Twenty-five percent of the population perishes from cancer."

Question: "How many cancer survivors are currently living in the United States?"
Answer: "Our best estimate at this time is 10.5 million."

2. **Realistically** How can such figures be ignored, even in a book of hope? Realism should not be depressing; it is to be stored in the recesses of the mind and accepted as an inevitable fate of all people. No one has ever left this earth alive—even astronauts plan to return.

3. **Mystically** To my surprise, many well-known persons have penned their ideas of death from unorthodox viewpoints. These views are presented here in no particular order. The reader's challenge is to decide whether these attitudes are too frivolous or if they awaken you to place death on a higher plane of acceptance.

This is the reader's challenge:

- Death—the last voyage, the longest, the best.

    — Thomas Wolfe
- If this is dying, I don't think much of it.

    —Lytton Strachey
- Death is nature's way of saying, "Your table is ready."

    —Robin Williams
- If you don't go to other people's funerals, they won't go to yours.

    —Unknown
- There are worse things than death for some people—take life, for instance.

    —Unknown
- Big deal! I'm used to dust.

    —Erma Bombeck
- In Heaven, all the interesting people are missing.

    —Freidrich Nietzsche
- There are worse things in life than death. Have you ever spent an evening with an insurance salesman?

    —Woody Allen
- No matter how rich you are, how famous or powerful you are, when you die the size of your funeral will depend on the weather.

    —Michael Pritchard

- For three days after death, hair and fingernails continue to grow but phone calls taper off.

—Johnny Carson

- It costs me never a stab or squirm to tread by chance upon a worm. "Aha, my little dear," I say, "your clan will pay me back some day."

—Dorothy Parker

Semantically, there is a difference between being "dead" and being "gone." Dead connotes forgotten, unthanked, erased from memory. Gone connotes remembered, brought to mind, and unforgettable.

Isn't that what life really is—a preparation of a dossier, or file, of remembrances for your loved ones, supporters, and acquaintances. Files differ in thickness. Review your file. Time abounds to add more pages as "gone" insurance.

So, you see that death can be inspirational after all!

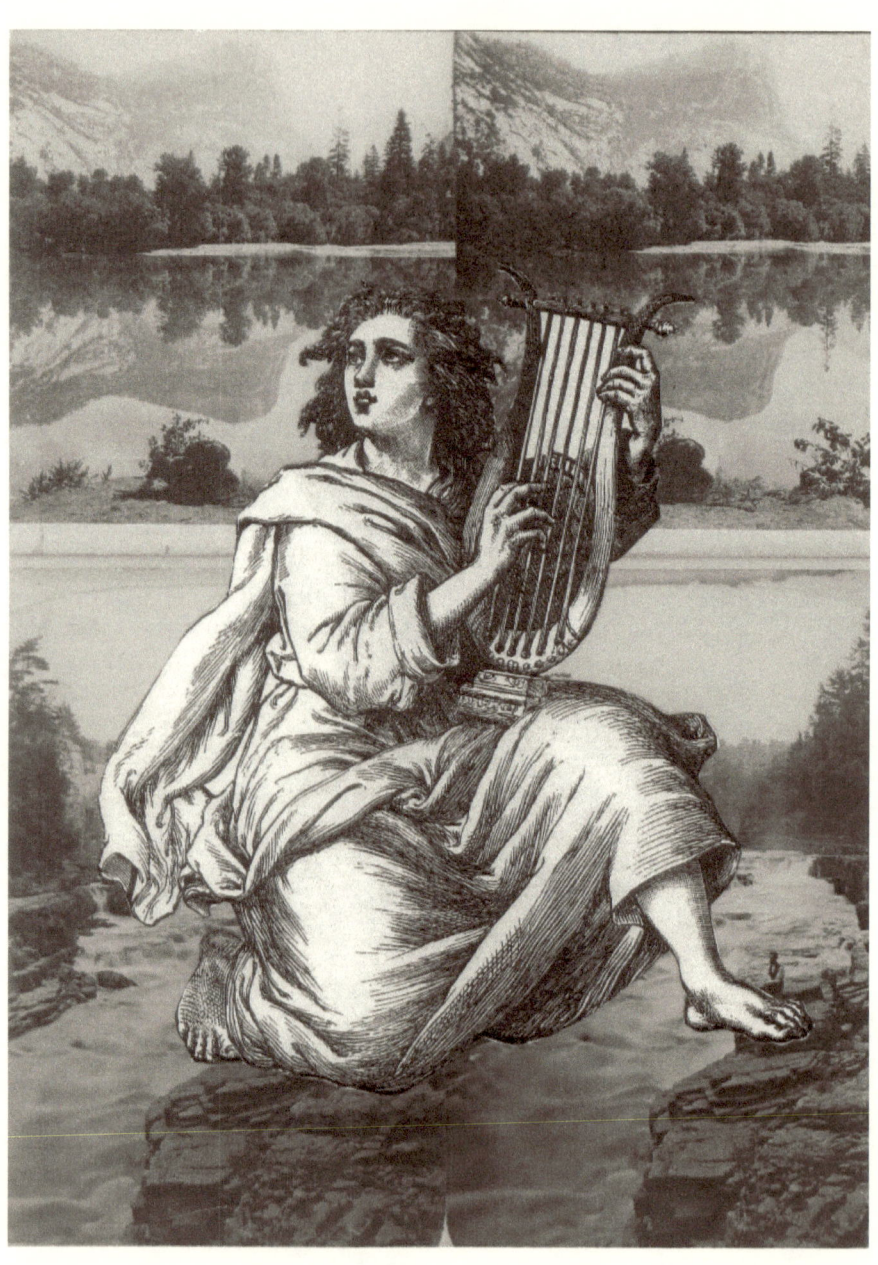

Chapter Fifteen

The Arms of Morpheus

The best bridge between despair and hope is a good
night's sleep.

—Unknown

To refresh your memory, Morpheus was the Greek goddess of sleep and dreams. For patients taking morphine, your drug name is derived from Morpheus.

Sleeping has been a challenge for me, and I assume that many fellow patients are faced with this nocturnal problem.

There is a joke about the person who stated, "I slept like a baby last night."

"How come?" said the friend.

"I wet my bed and cried all night," was the answer.

In this section, discussion will focus on strategies to assist the sleeping process:

- **Night-lights:** To prevent missteps or falling during the night, install 4- or 7- watt bulbs in appropriate electrical outlets.
- **Flashlight:** A flashlight is a vital appliance to place next to your bed. It should be used to accompany you to the bathroom or to locate medicines needed for administration.
- **Slipper socks:** Cold feet, a possible result of chemotherapy, can be disturbing at night. I have several pairs of slipper socks and find them quite reliable for bedtime use.
- **Small radio:** On the nights that Morpheus refuses to accept me into her arms for a period, I turn to a small battery-powered radio next to my bed. Turning it on at a low volume so as not to awaken my wife, I listen to an all-news station for the latest

bulletins. Sleep usually arrives in a short time—sometimes with the radio still on.

- **Book lights:** Should you wish to read during the periods when you are unable to sleep, book lights are available. They are battery equipped and attach to your book. I have one, and I am surprised how bright and handy it is.
- **Water bottle:** For dry or parched throats, a supply of bottled water should be available and convenient. I keep a one-liter bottle of commercially bought water next to my bed for nighttime sipping.
- **Sleep schedules:** Your sleeping hours may have changed from pre-illness days. I know mine have. I retire much earlier than before. My biological sleep clock has been severely altered. Becoming accustomed to new sleep schedules takes time and is directly related to the stress and chemotherapy aspects of the illness.
- **Oxygen:** Use your daytime hours to assure that all oxygen equipment is in proper working condition if needed during the night. Oxygen problems are not easily solved during nighttime hours when companies are closed.
- **Sleep medications:** Consult your oncologist should you feel the need for sleeping pills or additional pain medicines. Avoid over-the-counter products because they may conflict with the chemotherapy protocols chosen for you.
- **Suppers:** A question you must ask is the relationship of what you have for dinner and the effect it has on your sleep. Personally, I prefer light meals and very light dinners on the night before a chemo session. Experiment with your food intake, and it may contribute to a more productive sleep amount.

For those of us who struggle with the reward of a good night's sleep, keep up the search for answers. Finding strategies to enhance your sleeping is a lofty ambition, and the desire for improvement is inspirational. Shakespeare called it "a consummation devoutly to be wished."

END QUOTES

Sound sleep is the sleep you're in when it's time to get up.
—Unknown

The feeling of sleepiness when you are not in bed, and can't get there, is the meanest feeling in the world.
—Edgar Watson Howe

Etiquette is getting sleepy in public and not showing it.
—Hyman Maxwell Berston

Next to debt, the hardest thing to get out of is a warm bed on a cold morning.
—Unknown

Laugh and the world laughs with you, snore and you sleep alone.
—Anthony Burgess

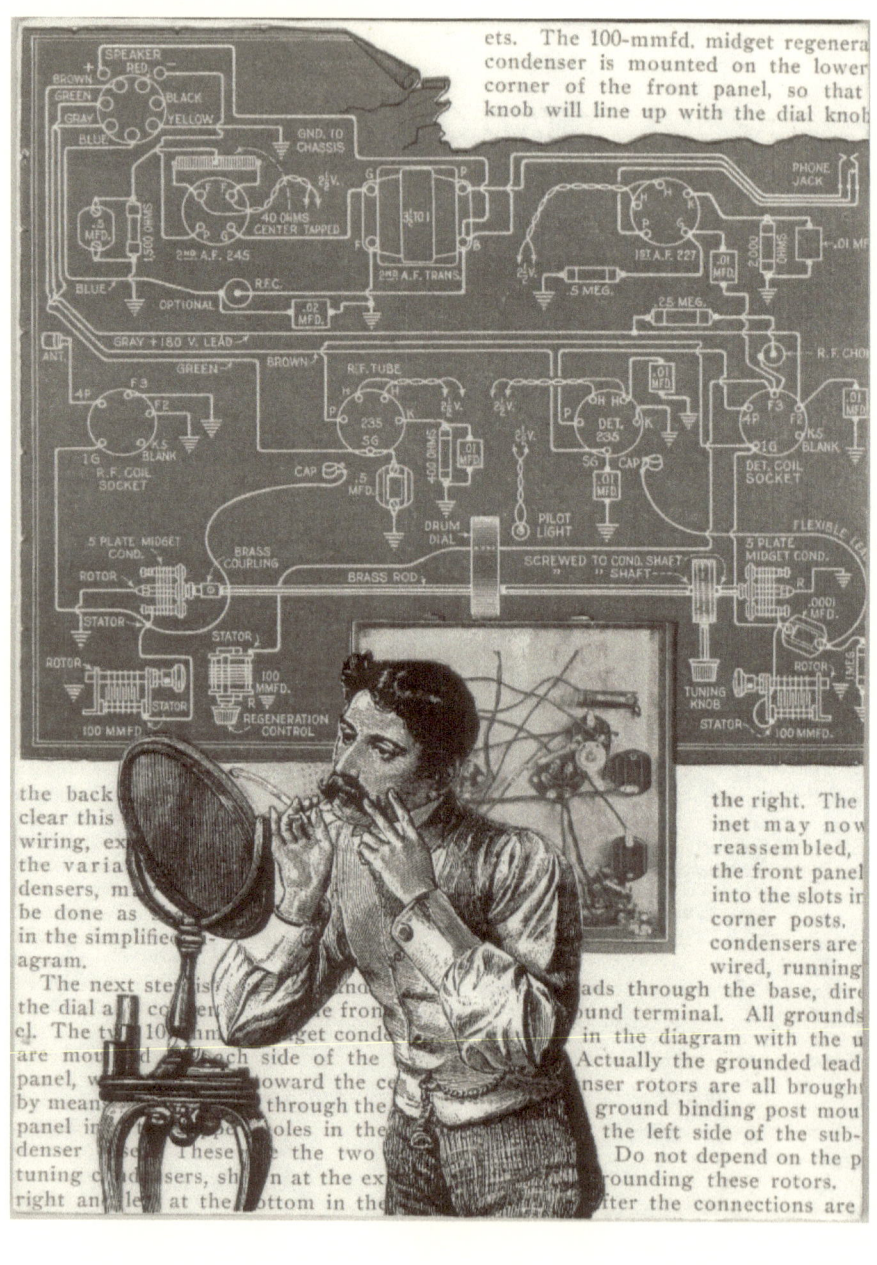

ets. The 100-mmfd. midget regenera
condenser is mounted on the lower
corner of the front panel, so that
knob will line up with the dial knob

the back
clear this
wiring, ex
the varia
densers, m
be done as
in the simplifie
agram.
   The next ste
the dial a
el. The t
are mo
panel, w
by mean
panel i
denser
tuning c
right an

the right. The
inet may now
reassembled,
the front panel
into the slots i
corner posts.
condensers are
wired, running
ads through the base, dire
und terminal. All grounds
in the diagram with the u
Actually the grounded lead
nser rotors are all brought
ground binding post mou
the left side of the sub-
Do not depend on the p
rounding these rotors.
fter the connections are

Chapter Sixteen

The Appearance of Men

Don't blame the mirror if your face is faulty.
—Nikolai Gogol

Are male patients inclined to be less concerned about their appearance and personal hygiene than they should? This section offers male patients strategies for improving their appearance.

- **Shaving:** Electric shavers make the morning shave less horrendous. If assistance is needed, the shaver is easily used and completes the job without the stress and strain of soap and razor. For patients on blood thinners, there is a safety factor when a razor is used.
- **Showering:** This can be an area of concern when weakness or a balance problem is present. Some men may feel squeamish or reluctant to have a female health aide assist in the shower process. For these men, select a male health aide who will assist in the process. You may wish to reserve the washing of private parts and rectal areas as your own province. A shower chair is an excellent appliance to conserve strength. Again, I use mine extensively. A plastic shower mat is added insurance to prevent loss of balance or slipping upon entering or exiting the shower area.
- **Bathing:** The tub bath is an excellent source of relaxation and comfort. However entering and exiting the tub may cause problems. Assistance may be required to negotiate the process.
- **Teeth:** Morning and evening brushing is mandatory. Bridges and false teeth must be kept clean and stored overnight in proper receptacles. Should mouth and/or gum sores develop because of chemotherapy, notify your oncologist for soothing medications.
- **Nails:** Fingernails and toenails should be trimmed periodically. Assistance may be required to manipulate the clippers—especially

the toenails. Keep your fingernails clean and use an antibacterial soap for washing hands.

- **Port:** Many cancer patients have a chest port as an aid to receiving chemotherapy. Should irritation or pain occur at this location, notify your oncologist or medical team.
- **Clothing:** Shakespeare said, "The apparel oft proclaims the man." To what extent should a male cancer patient allow the illness to affect his outward appearance negatively? Can an acceptable level of dress and fashion be brokered? I think so.

Be sensitive to odors! Socks and underwear must smell clean and be changed daily. Being odorific is not a pleasant way of entering a room.

Clothes should be cleaned to present a tidy presentation—not overdressed but appropriate for the situation. In no way am I suggesting that male patients should step out of the pages of *Esquire* or *Gentleman's Quarterly*. However, there are substandard appearances that could be avoided with a little care.

Looking good, feeling better!

END QUOTES

They should put expiration dates on clothes so we would know when they go out of style.

—Garry Shandling

A man can wear a hat for years without being oppressed by its shabbiness.

—James Douglas

I should warn you that underneath these clothes I'm wearing boxer shorts and I know how to use them.

—Robert Orben

A fair exterior is a silent recommendation.

—Syrus

The world is a looking glass and gives back to every man the reflection of his own face.

—William Makepeace Thackeray

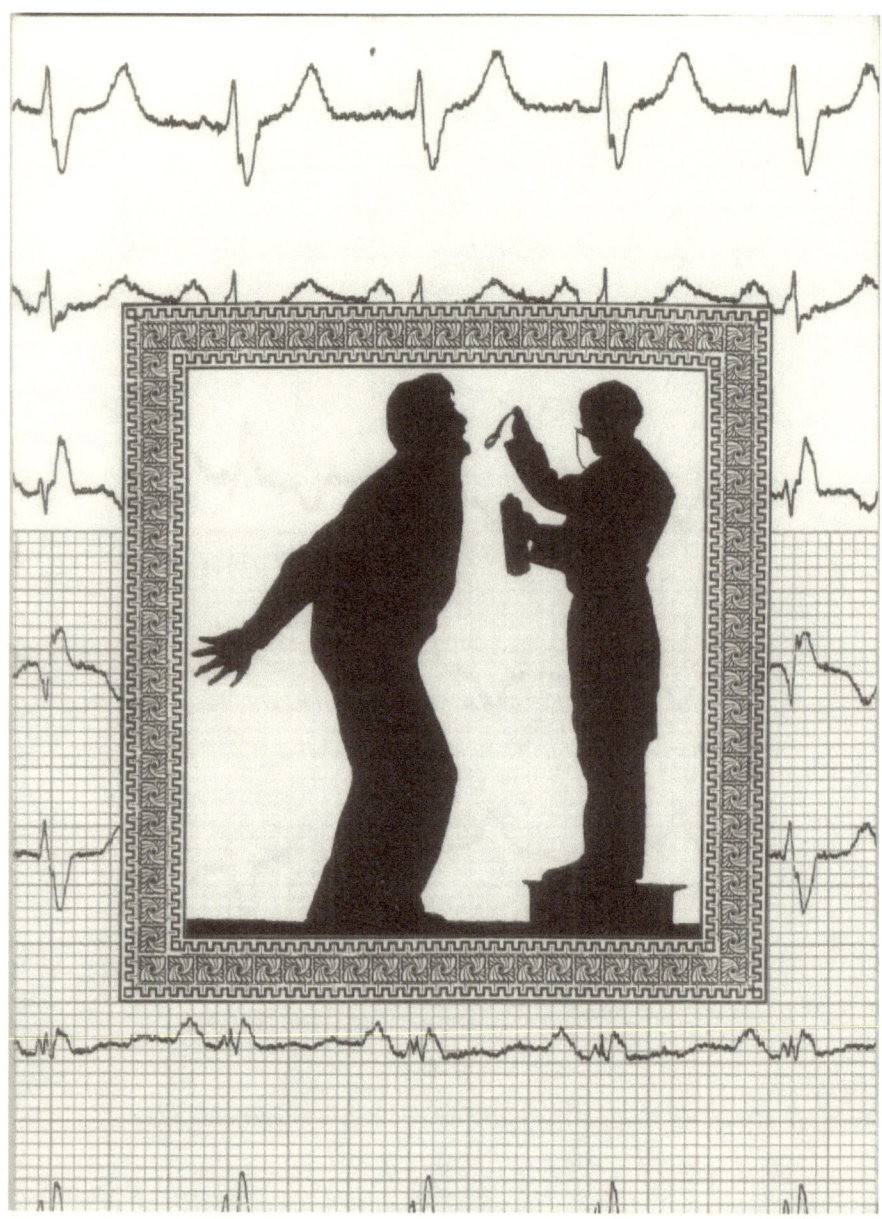

Chapter Seventeen

The Difficult Patient

No one can be reasonable and angry at the same time.

—Unknown

The oncology medical office and the chemotherapy domicile appear to be a microcosm of society. Into its environs spill segments of society from all corners of our population. The range of reactions from this group covers a wide area of responses.

Of particular concern in this section is the difficult patient— one whose agitation and annoyance are unmasked.

Does the medical office waiting room bring out the worst in patients? Likewise, is this true for the hematology-testing lab?

Through the years, I have observed that cats enjoy rubbing their furry flanks against table legs, sofas, or pants legs. Cats appear to thrive on friction.

Could this be true for a segment of our population?

If this is so, it is an extravagant waste of energy that could be employed in more positive channels.

To carry this one step further, are there people who possess "short fuses"? Cancer patients are people too, and many reflect these attitudes.

WAITING TIME

The medical waiting room does not run on airport time. Delays are prevalent and expected. Due to this, I have witnessed hostile and antagonistic situations. Many patients exhibit inflexibility and outward irritation at their medical teams. Patience must be developed and used to replace anger. Stress reduction is essential for positive thinking.

ORGANIZATIONAL STRATEGIES

The difficult patient lacks structure and a system of record keeping. Frustration abounds when appointments are missed, dates are forgotten, and test results are misplaced. All of these things can result in adverse emotional reactions.

Calendar confusion is quite distressing. To correct this situation, meet with your medical team to acquire one of the calendars supplied by a drug company. Your team will organize your calendar to ensure date verification.

It is the responsibility of the cancer patient to improve the "chemistry" between team and patient. Agitation is a severe form of self-punishment! Do not thrive on controversy.

END QUOTES

Anger is just one letter short of <u>danger</u>.

—Unknown

Grow angry slowly—there's plenty of time.

—Ralph Waldo Emerson

Anger makes your mouth work faster than your mind.

—Unknown

The best remedy for a short temper is a long walk.

—Jacqueline Schiff

Don't hate, it's too big a burden to bear.

—Dr. Martin Luther King, Jr.

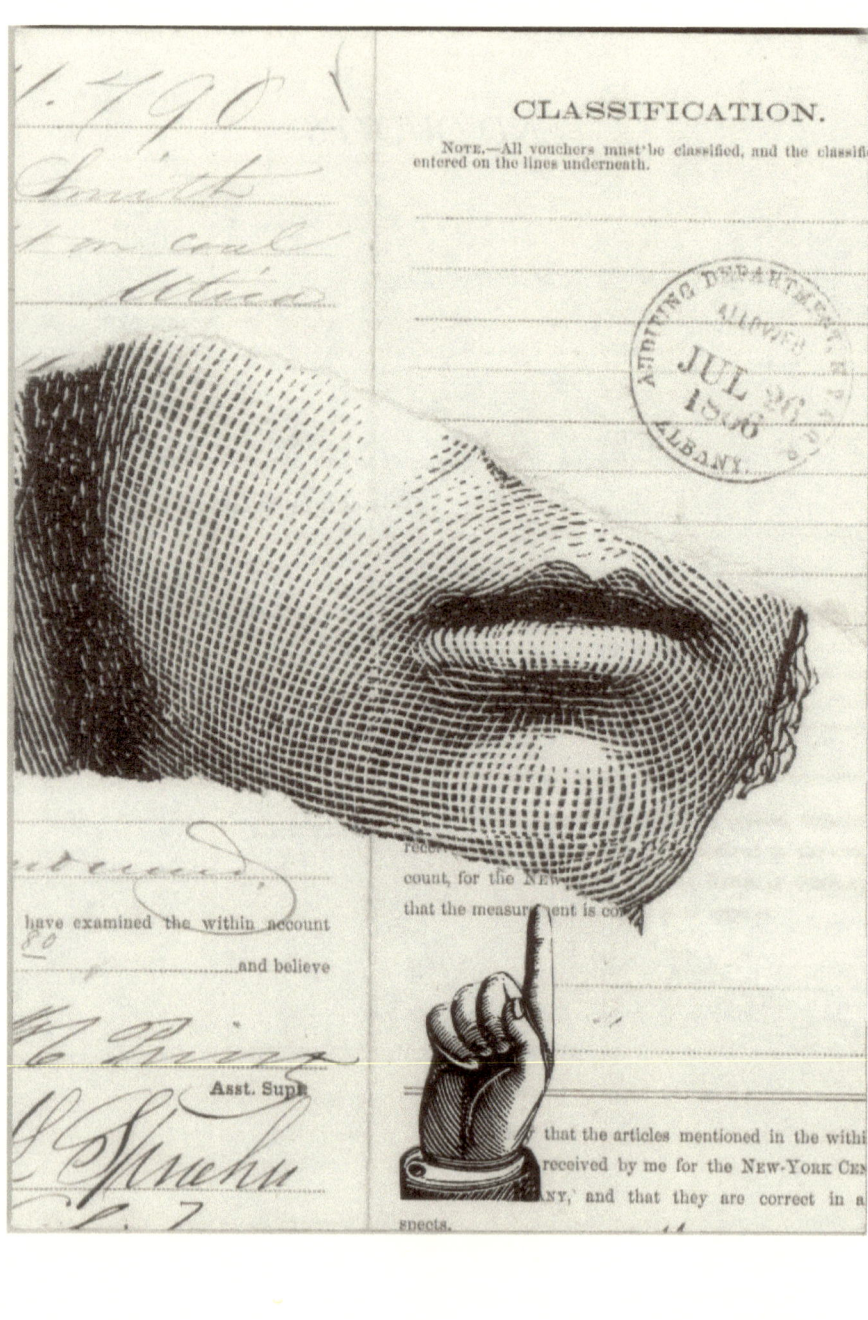

Chapter Eighteen

Directed Speech

The less you talk, the more you're listened to.
—*Abigail Van Buren*

It is essential that a "free flow" of communication exists between the medical team, oncologist, and the cancer patient. This exchange contributes significantly to the dignity and pride of the patient. A patient's active participation in the decision-making process is essential.

Planning strategies, test results, and protocol changes are all part of this process.

However, caregivers and family supporters should be alert to a patient's growing difficulty in continuing to participate in the sharing process. Factors limiting participation may include the cancer's advanced stages, the patient's age, inability to focus, and loss of lucidity.

Should this happen, decisions by a family advocate or a family representative should become more prominent, and a more direct role can be advanced. Done tactfully and without loss of dignity, speech is directed to the family advocate who assumes the role of decision maker.

Once again, I would like to reiterate that this matter is quite delicate and emotional. Exercise sensitivity in this role "takeover" to minimize its emotional impact on the cancer patient. The degree of intercession is a family decision to be reached by consensus. Above all, afford the patient a sympathetic chord.

Respect is never compromised! Your loved one is still the same person and is due the same courtesy and civility as before. Being mindful of the past will ensure a more tolerant and obliging attitude toward your loved one.

Shakespeare called it the "milk of human kindness." The compassion of the family advocate or representative exhibits this goodness.

END QUOTES

If you don't say anything, you won't be called to repeat it.
—Calvin Coolidge

The louder he talked about his honor, the faster we counted our spoons.
—Ralph Waldo Emerson

Speak when you are angry and you will make the best speech you will ever regret.
—Ambrose Bierce

Talk to a man about himself, and he will listen for hours.
—Benjamin Disraeli

Wisdom is the reward you get for a lifetime of listening when you preferred to talk.
—Doug Larson

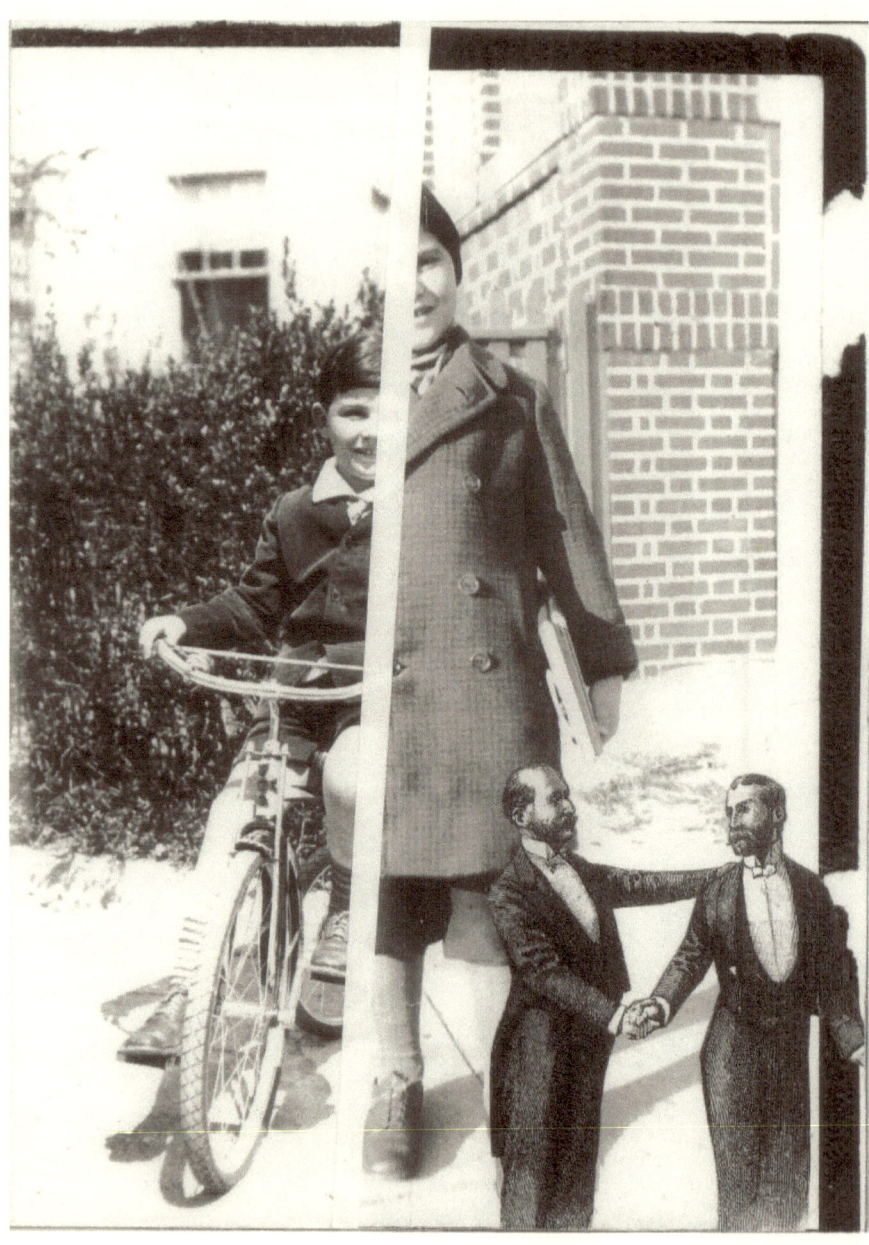

Chapter Nineteen

Mending Wall

The more a man knows, the more he forgives.
—*Catherine the Great*

Robert Frost, the eminent New England poet, captures the essence of hostility and imprisonment in his poem "Mending Wall." The poem focuses on the handcrafted stone walls that separate Vermont homesteads and designate boundary lines. Frost notices that one of his stone walls has been breached—with the stones scattered along the ground.

As the poet walks over to the damaged wall, he notices his neighbor busily replacing the stones and mending the wall. Frost questions the need for such fences because he is "walling in as well as walling out." The neighbor replies, "Good fences make good neighbors." The neighbor has created an atmosphere of isolation and noncommunication with the poet.

In this chapter, the reader will discuss barriers or hindrances for the development of positive relationships with family, siblings, supporters, and the medical team. The barriers in question are grudges, estrangement, and general dislike for relatives or acquaintances.

The negatives of bearing grudges are obvious. The emotional erosion and the festering hatred sours the spirit and poisons the soul.

Grudges evolve from many sources. An insult, malicious gossip, financial misconducts, and spiteful actions all contribute to grudge formation. Ruthless and vicious actions may also affect your relationships.

If there ever was a time in your life to repair "fractured" relationships, the onset of cancer-related illness provides an ideal impetus. Cancer is an entry card into the area of forgiveness. Mending relationships is not an easy task. However, cancer can enable you to take those steps necessary for attitude readjustment.

How deep is your hurt? Is it so deep that forgiveness is out of the question? Perhaps time has elapsed and the causes have become blurred and can be wiped away with the tears of time. Explore the healing properties of time. For some, they can forgive but not forget. For others, "wiping the slate clean" may require exhaustive efforts.

The popular expression "to bury the hatchet" has a pertinent origin. The American Indian practiced a native custom of a ceremonial burial of a war weapon as a signal that a war had ended. Reconciling family estrangements is a modified version of a ceremonial burial of grudges.

What replaces the anger you have felt over the cause of your resentment? The answer is forgiveness. It is a gift you are bestowing—the gift of giving. Presidents and governors grant pardons. Could not this gesture be extended to siblings, relatives, and acquaintances?

We know that a *don*ation is a grant or a philanthropic gift. A par*don* refers to forgiveness, while con*done* is to free from blame. Something that is unpar*don*able is inexcusable. Your pardon is a peace effort to "pocket the affront." Granting amnesty is a modified form of exoneration—wiping the slate clean.

Poet Milton Kaplan compares hatred to a growing tumor deep in the convolutions of the brain. Cancer, too, grows deep inside the caverns of the body. Although bearing grudges may be a nonmalignant form of cancer, it too gnaws away at life-giving sources of energy.

Forgiveness is not a loss of control over your feelings. In fact, it will intensify your desire to survive. Frictions, long festering, will be surrendered and replaced with positive actions. How, then, can you put closure on a hurtful period of life?

BREAKING THE ICE

- *A phone call*—Surely the most direct and convenient way of reestablishing relations with friends, family, and colleagues.
- *A greeting card*—A visit to your local card store will reveal a plethora of cards for every occasion. Cards celebrate and recognize accomplishments, milestones, and happy events.
- *A personal letter*—A handwritten letter is a very effective icebreaker. You may wish to discuss your illness through the use of metaphors, such as, "The grass has not been too green for me lately," or "the sun has not been shining too brightly on me," or "I'm trying to turn stormy days into beautiful weather."
- *The holidays*—Christmas, New Year's, Easter, Thanksgiving, Chanukah, and Kwanzaa set the stage for a card or phone call as a peace offering.

Call it "turning the other cheek" or anything else that signifies a cessation of hostilities. The time has come to "mend" the shards of broken relations. Your illness will provide the glue to repair the damage.

END QUOTES

We love without reason, and without reason we hate.
—Jean-Francois Reynard

To err is human; to forgive, divine.
—Alexander Pope

He who cannot forgive others destroys the bridge over which he himself must pass.
—George Herbert

The stupid neither forgive nor forget, the naïve forgive and forget, the wise forgive but do not forget.
—Thomas Szasz

Forgiving and being forgiven are two names for the same thing. The important thing is that a discord has been resolved.
—C. S. Lewis

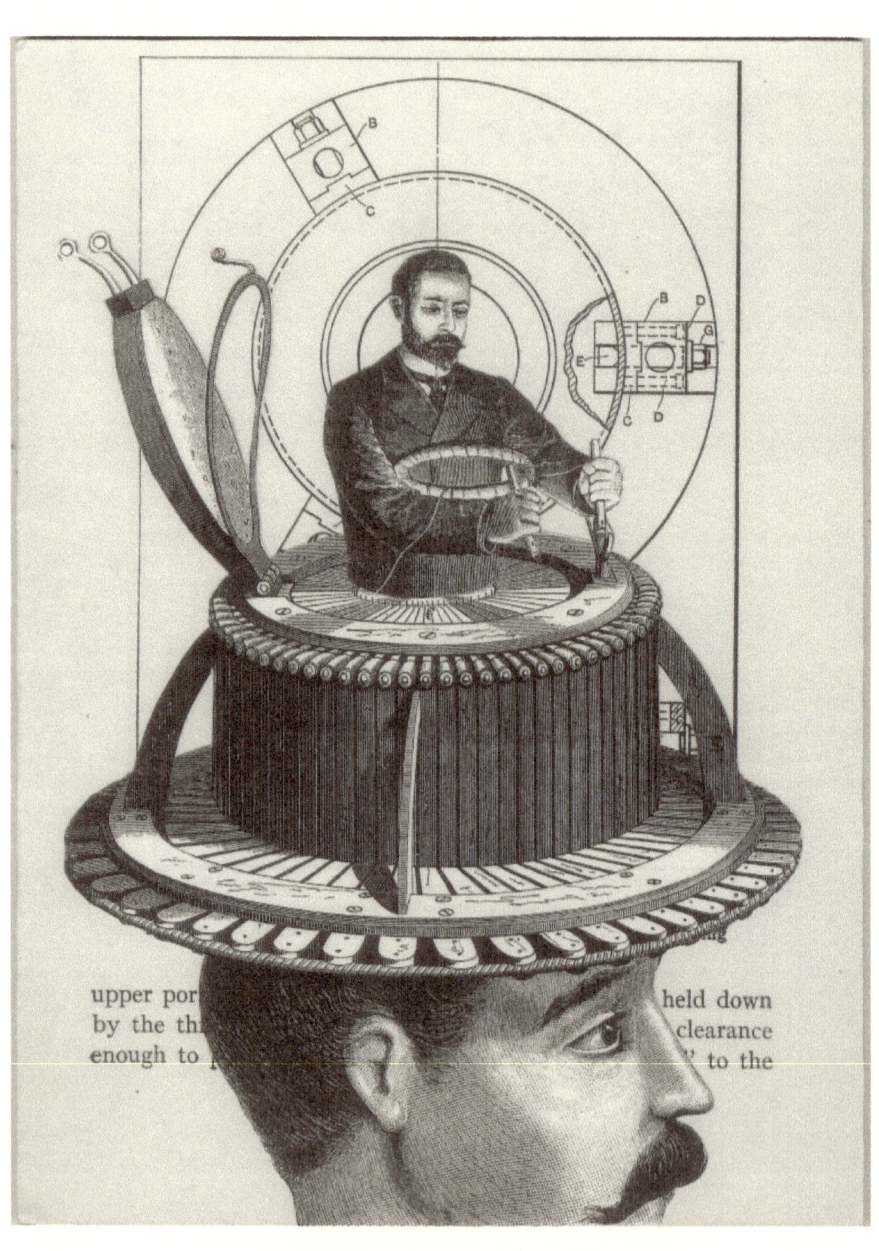

upper por held down
by the th clearance
enough to to the

Chapter Twenty

Controlling Control

The hardest thing to give is IN.

—*Unknown*

The word *control* is a term used to describe the degree of dominance a person has over his or her daily affairs.

Control indicates power, influence, and independence. It is ego gratifying and provides status and emotional security.

On the other hand, loss of control is a complex and unhealthy event. Its effects can be devastating for persons who have become accustomed to having the upper hand.

The question here is, "Does a diagnosis of cancer bring with it a loss of control for the individual?" Furthermore, does cancer pull the rug out from under the pillars of dominance that many people enjoy prior to their illness?

Unfortunately, those individuals who had stature, prominence, and authority are in for a rude awakening. They will discover that they must now share control, and that compromise, cooperation, and restraint will become their goals.

Loss of control can be an ego-shattering experience. However, by substituting coexistence and partnerships with supporters and a medical team, dependency does not have to be a fearful experience. Control disputes are nonproductive and emotionally destructive. Cancer patients must learn to accept their new dependency as a survival mechanism. Shared control is a goal that deserves immediate attention.

Loss of control has physical as well as emotional implications. The disease may affect control over balance, walking, sleeping, driving, and working conditions. I have found that control over mobility has been altered. Walking is done at a much slower pace. There is a fear factor regarding falling and loss of balance. Dressing and undressing takes much longer. And so you see that priorities have changed.

The "priority of perfection" has been altered and replaced with the priority of remission. Letting go of the insignificant frees you to concentrate on regaining your health.

STRATEGIES FOR SURVIVAL

Walking

There are times that a simple walk from the car to the mall entrance may be filled with pitfalls. Before commencing your walk, survey the area. Be alert to potential problem areas such as high curbs, pavement cracks, and areas that present problems for wheelchairs and walkers. Watch the flow of traffic and utilize the handicap spaces if you have the required permit.

Driving

Consult your oncologist and medical team for their consent before you resume driving. In addition, several factors are worth considering:

- Are you taking any medications that may affect your reaction time?
- Is your vision and perception of distances acceptable?
- Do you have a cell phone available for emergencies?
- Can you enter and exit your vehicle unaided and without difficulty?
- Is your cane, walker, or wheelchair accessible?
- If your car has not been used for a while, have you checked the fuel and oil indicators on the dashboard?

Time

For many cancer patients, they have entered a new dimension. Time moves more slowly. Pacing is slower. Movements are choreographed and appear in slow motion. Everything we do is different from what we did prior to the diagnosis. The past becomes the standard by which we measure the present.

Working

For those patients who are working, inform your employer about your ability to perform tasks at a pre-illness speed. Your rights are protected by state and federal regulations. Employers should be empathetic for employees who are working despite their cancer obligations.

You can handle tasks at home with greater facility if you break them down or reorganize them into smaller segments. Reduce the complexity of tasks. They may require longer time to complete, and they may also be mentally and/or physically draining.

Sharing control was the theme of this chapter. I recall seeing a television remote control for the first time. It puzzled me that this new device would replace the direct control that viewers had over their television sets. No more knobs to adjust, switches to turn off and on, and dials to reset. Control was being refocused, shared, and improved.

Do you get the message? Just like "sharing control."

END QUOTES

Few burdens are heavy when everybody lifts.

—Unknown

The unending problem of growing old was not how he changed, but how things did.

—Toni Morrison

You're either part of the solution, or you're part of the problem.

—Eldridge Cleaver

Men talk of killing time, while time kills them.

—Dion Boucicault

If there is anything small, shallow, or ugly about a person, giving him a little authority will bring it out.

—Unknown

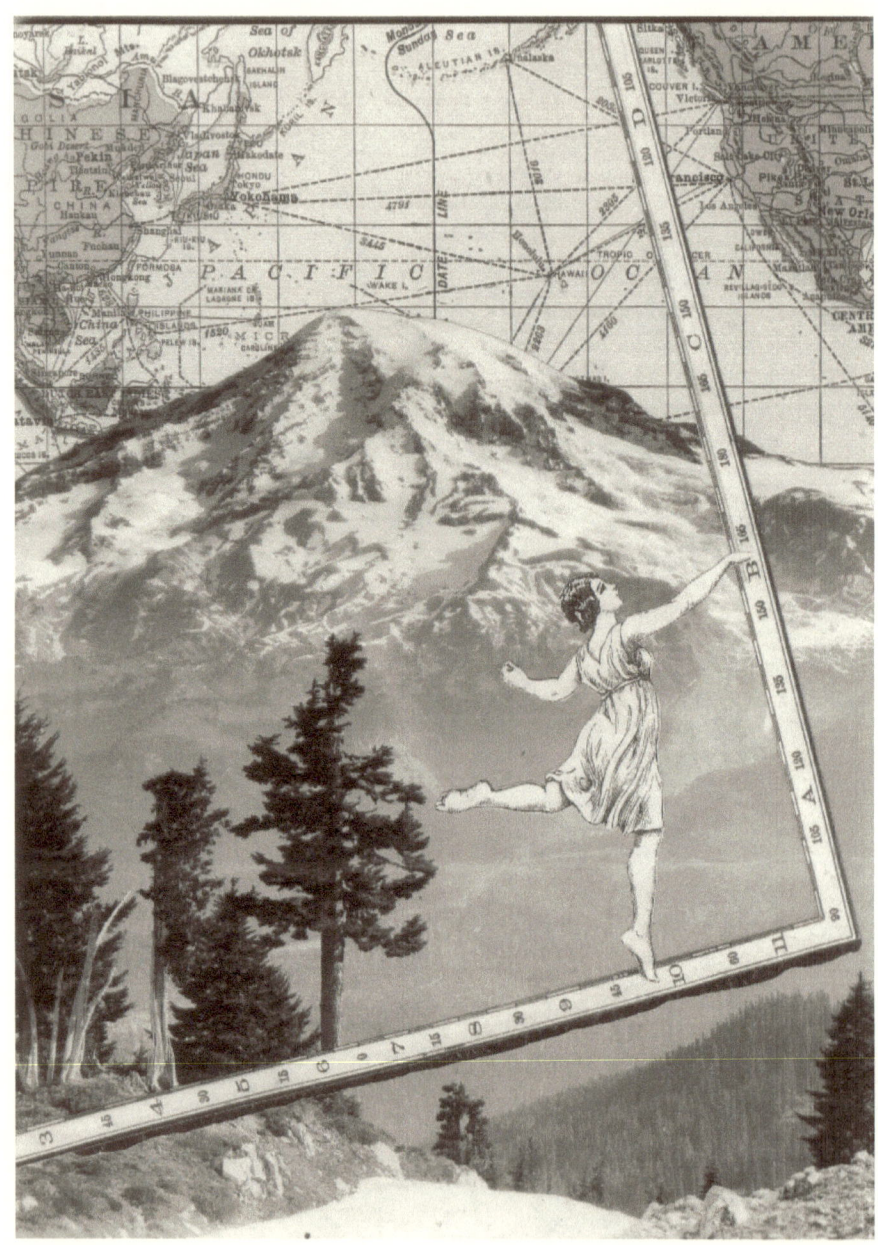

Chapter Twenty-One

Unfulfilled Dreams

Nothing happens unless first a dream.

—*Carl Sandburg*

Shakespeare called a dream an "airy nothing," but it is much more than that. Your visions, goals, and aspirations are valuable adjuncts on your road to recovery.

Your vision or dream of recovery is *not* an "airy nothing." A driving force, it compels you to take medications and undergo chemo and radiation. A dream is hardly a deluded belief or a form of self-deception. Your dream is real and well within reach.

Does cancer inhibit visions or dreams of the future?

Undoubtedly, the physical or mental restrictions imposed by your particular type of cancer may impose restrictions on your ability to fulfill dreams and wishes. Dreams may have to be tailored to your needs, but certainly not abandoned.

Your hopes for a better tomorrow take many forms. These hopes are diverse and will require strategies for fulfillment new to your lifestyle.

Unlike Don Quixote, the hero of *Man of La Mancha,* your quest is *not* an impossible dream. The strategies that will be presented here are offered with ease of accomplishment. These strategies will bring your dreams within reach.

Specifically, this chapter will explore alternate means to satisfy your thirst for travel, knowledge, serenity, and exploration. The stress is on "alternate means," due to the effects of chemo and/or radiation on your stamina and energy level.

LITERATURE

Cancer does not have to prevent expansion of your literary mind. Individualized reading is an experience that has countless benefits. If done in your comfort zone, and providing that your aches and pains do not interrupt the flow between author and reader, I recommend the reading habit.

Reading is a path to self-discovery. You can see how others have met similar challenges and conquered them. You can see what drives and motivates people to surmount difficult tasks. In addition, self-discovery helps you to see yourself more clearly by identifying with the characters you are visualizing.

Reading is also a means of "living vicariously." Mountain climbing, deep-sea exploration, and jungle treks can be digested while sitting in a comfortable armchair. The four corners of the world are within easy reach through the magic pages of travel essays. Furthermore, reading is a means of enjoying the beauty of language—the phrases and descriptions used by authors to describe their actions. This beauty provides an escape mechanism by contrasting the beauty of language with the unpleasantness of disease.

The unpleasantness referred to may be nausea, fatigue, or lack of concentration—fostered by your medications. If so, adjust your reading strategies.

One novel approach (no pun intended) is to utilize a collection of book summaries, such as *The Novel 100,* by Daniel S. Burt, published in 2004. It contains the plot outlines of one hundred classics. In similar fashion, there is *Plot Outlines of 100 Famous Plays,* by Van H. Cartnell.

Reading summaries of classic novels and plays is not surrendering to mediocrity. It is an acceptable method of convenience and moderation. Summaries will provide enlightenment and, if your health permits, develop an appetite to read the original work in its entirety.

You can satisfy your lust for learning by altering your reading style. Rather than lamenting and grieving for your past powers of concentration, reconstruct your reading habits in alignment with energy levels.

TRAVEL

Poet John Masefield called his desire to travel "a fire in my heels." The yearning to see the world may exist undiminished in the soul of the cancer patient. While mobility restrictions inhibit loftier ambitions, travel may still be within your reach— with the approval of your oncologist. Special attention must be given to available medical services, walking distances, wheelchair and walker accessibility, and sleeping accommodations. Perhaps a handicapped facility would be in order.

CRUISES

For the uninitiated, cruise ships are "floating hotels." These ocean liners are sanitary, superbly comfortable, and luxurious in design. If your dream is sailing on a magnificent cruise ship, employ strategies to assure a successful trip.

First, your oncologist will determine if your present condition allows such an undertaking. Second, a travel agent should be utilized to secure accommodations in consonance with your health needs. Special attention must be given to cabin location, proximity to elevators, and cabin size. Naturally, single occupancy is always more expensive than double occupancy.

Poet John Keats called the sea a "feast for tired eyes." If you are enamored with the smell of salt air and the gentle rocking of ocean swells, I recommend a balcony or veranda as part of your cabin selection.

Questions for your travel agent should include the following:

- *Will dietary restrictions be honored?*
- *Are the medical facilities adequate?*
- *Is the ship wheelchair accessible?*
- *Is there a library aboard (if you enjoy reading)?*
- *Are there abundant elevators?*
- *Is there a stall shower in the cabin?*

Last but not least, inquire about insurance for trip cancellation or interruption. Fortunately for me, my insurance for trip interruption was utilized when I was diagnosed with lung cancer several days after my cruise ended.

Should you desire to remain on board for your entire cruise, or take all meals in your cabin, that is easily arranged. Optional travel arrangements are never compulsory, and provisions are always made for passengers who choose not to leave the ship.

TRAIN TRAVEL

The lure of the rails may be just as strong as your sea fever. However, it would be a mistake to compare rail and cruise travel. The mesmerizing effects of the swaying cars as they amble down the tracks can have a salubrious influence on insomnia. Train travel is in miniature, with everything on a smaller scale, tailored to fit the restrictions of limited space.

Train travel is a panoply of ever-changing scenery. The beauty of our country or neighboring Canada flashes by in a constant stream. Majestic mountains, winding rivers, steep gorges, and fertile fields offer an uncompromised display of unforgettable views.

Passenger fellowship is rampant. Friendships are easily made from the assemblage of travelers. Even the most recalcitrant traveler finds himself part of the group.

The glass-enclosed observation car offers an unobstructed view of the passing scene from the comfort of spacious armchairs. For patients with restrictive mobility, the observation car offers a grand opportunity for sightseeing.

Before any commitment with your travel agent, please pose the following questions:

- *Will my compartment have bathroom facilities?*
- *If my compartment lacks bathroom facilities, what provisions are provided, and where are they located?*
- *How accessible is the dining car from my compartment?*
- *Are the sleeping accommodations satisfactory for a person with health concerns?*
- *What provisions are made for luggage and personal possessions?*
- *Can a wheelchair or walker fit inside the compartment?*
- *Do the passageways have handrails to assist people with walking difficulties?*
- *Are meals included in the price of the journey?*
- *Is an insurance policy available for the trip?*
- *Will taxis be available at train stops along the way?*

MUSIC

Consider the possibility of broadening your base of musical knowledge. The thirst for increasing your curiosity about the world of music can be satisfied quite easily. My lofty ambitions in this area focus on classical and contemporary compositions of our greatest composers.

Using tapes and/or CDs or an iPod, I let the music wash over me in therapeutic waves. With the volume turned up to a comfortable level, reclining on a nearby sofa, I enjoy the strains of classical efforts without commercial interruptions. With an iPod, you can custom create the contents. Although the effect of music on cancer remission has never been confirmed, it is certainly worth a try. I look forward to my daily bouts of music appreciation—a rewarding and relaxing interlude.

Borders and Barnes & Noble bookstores have a voluminous number of tapes and CDs at popular prices to cater to all musical tastes.

If your dream is to increase your base knowledge of the world of music, start your journey without restriction. With your eyes closed, and visualizing the symphonic orchestra, escape from the tedium of daily routines is immediate. Undoubtedly, music soothes and satisfies basic instincts. Musical interludes, regardless of genre, refresh and revitalize the spirit. Cancer patients certainly can profit from a renascence of the spirit.

EXPLORATION

Ali Baba had his magic carpet to explore and discover untold riches. For us, there is no magic carpet, but with a little imagination, you can introduce into your daily existence strategies that simulate the magic carpet.

TRAVEL JOURNALISTS

Your neighborhood bookstores have shelves abundant with books—not travel guides—that explore every region of our globe. The six major travel journalists that come to mind as first-class writers are Paul Theroux, Bill Bryson, Jon Krakauer, Frances Mayes, Jason Roberts, and Peter Mayle. Their books are adventuresome and captivating as they skirt the world, discovering places most people long to visit.

From the comfort of your easy chair, your desire to explore can be fulfilled without a magic carpet.

TRAVEL HOSTS

Travel programs on public television, cable, and high-definition (HDTV) television appear on a daily basis. The hosts of these travel programs are knowledgeable, cordial, and dedicated to the pursuit of discovery. Become familiar with the names of the major hosts: Rudy Maxa, Rick Steves of PBS, Samantha Brown of the Travel Channel, Michael Palin, Anthony Bourdain, and Andrew Zimmern.

Naturally, you will have to check your local TV listings for the day, time, and channel for the multitude of travel programs. From your easy chair, the far sections of the globe are as close as your remote.

Bon voyage and happy travel are devout wishes as you explore and discover new meanings of life.

AUDIOBOOKS

Should your illness prevent reading directly from books, or should your energy level be below an acceptable point, audiobooks may be a viable alternative. Fiction, nonfiction, romance, and mystery are available, including the classics.

Most bookstores have an incredibly large collection of audiobooks. Also check with your public library to see if audiobooks are available for circulation.

Some cancer patients have mentioned that having someone read to them helps the sleeping process. Isn't it worth a try?

ACCEPTING THE VICARIOUS

For many cancer patients, firsthand experiences may be out of the question or, at best, placed on the back burner for a while. The stamina and physical dexterity needed to experience the joys of land travel, ocean cruises, or train journeys may not be present.

Vicarious pursuit of dreams and wishes is well within your reach. The travel journalists, hosts, and media specialists provide a wondrous opportunity to see the world from your bed, armchair, or sofa. The new high-definition TV presents an uncannily realistic portrayal of travel scenery. Vibrant colors and three-dimensional views transport the viewer to foreign shores.

Your magic carpet is calling you to step aboard. Have a good flight!

END QUOTES

Few wishes come true by themselves.

—June Smith

Hold fast to dreams, for if dreams die, life is a broken-winged bird that cannot fly.

—Langston Hughes

The most important things in life aren't things.

—Unknown

Walk on, walk on, with hope in your heart; and you'll never walk alone.

—Oscar Hammerstein II

Don't be unhappy if your dreams never come true—just be thankful your nightmares don't.

—Unknown

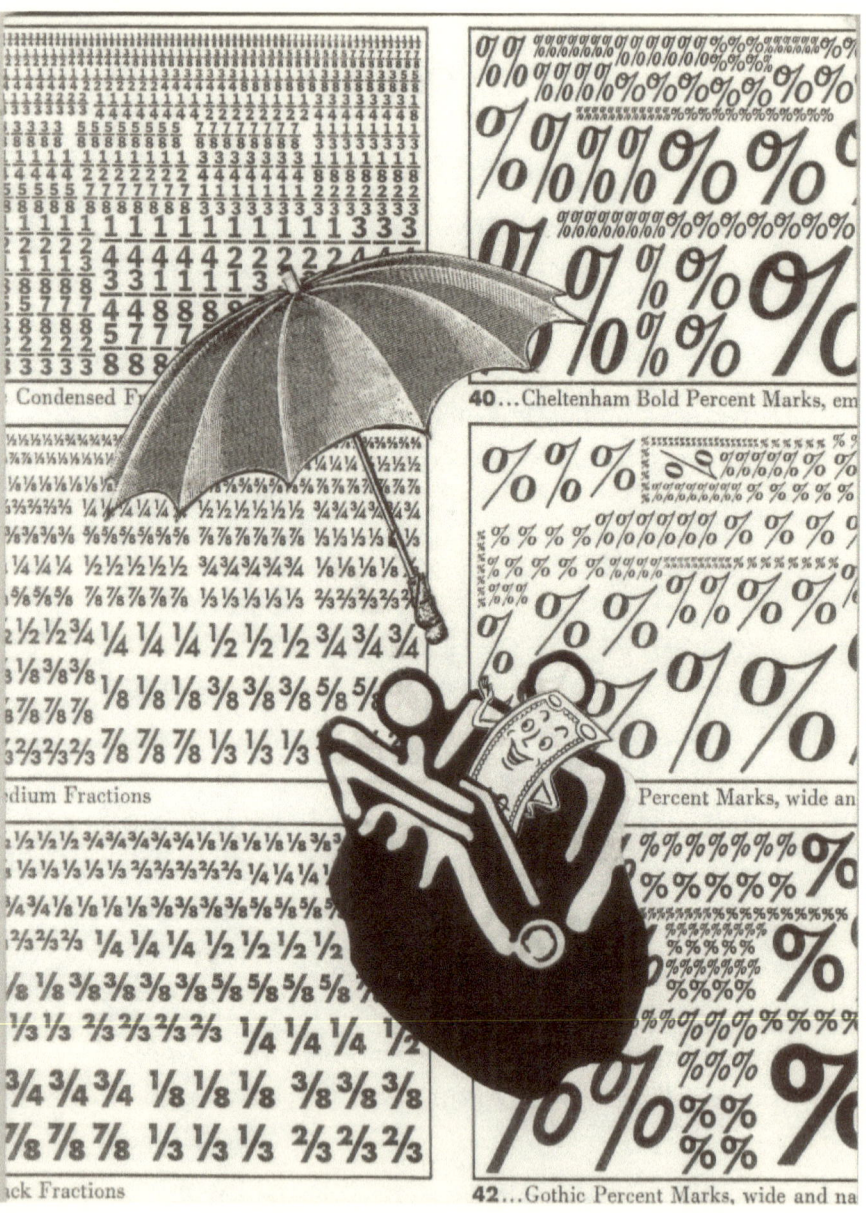

Condensed F...

40...Cheltenham Bold Percent Marks, em...

Medium Fractions

Percent Marks, wide an...

...ack Fractions

42...Gothic Percent Marks, wide and na...

Chapter Twenty-Two

Releasing Purse Strings

The miracle is this—the more we share, the more
we have.

—*Leonard Nimoy*

Not only does cancer inflict disastrous physical damage to the body, but it also causes complex and far-reaching episodes to economic and financial reserves. In addition, rising gas prices at the pump and consumer prices at the market have all contributed to draining financial resources.

Whether it is corporate greed or lack of governmental controls, your personal treasury is under siege. The outflow of funds must be adequate to meet obligations, thus avoiding arrears.

Cancer knows no boundaries and financial exemptions. It can ravage the industrialist as well as the sales associate, the financier as well as the maintenance worker. The financial obligations instigated by cancer can become overwhelming if not catastrophic. Fortunately, Medicare, HMOs, and insurance plans may serve to ease the burdens imposed by the sickness.

My experiences with HMO and Medicare have been excellent and stress reducing. I have not fallen behind on accounts payable, and I do not find myself lacking the essentials of daily living.

To expand on the theme of this chapter, "Releasing Purse Strings," it is convenient to divide cancer patients into three groups:

Group A	Cancer patients who are financially secure
Group B	Cancer patients who are financially sufficient, and able to meet obligations
Group C	Cancer patients who are financially inadequate with funds in short supply

In summary, the three As define the picture: Group A—affluent; Group B—adequate; Group C—arrears. Our focus in this chapter is the influence Group A can have on Group C. We will also explore cancer as an exponent of generosity and goodwill.

Financial resources are dependent on the familial structure and organization. This structure reflects complexity by its very nature:

- Single mom with cancer, still working
- Single dad with cancer, still working
- Single mom with cancer, not working
- Single dad with cancer, not working
- Couple, both working, one with cancer
- Couple, one working, one with cancer
- Retired couple, one working, one with cancer
- Retired couple, not working, one with cancer
- Retired couple, both with cancer, not working
- Single retired person, with cancer, not working

Income from salaries, pensions, annuities, IRA distributions, stocks, bonds, and mutual funds also contribute to the financial "health" of the family unit.

It is not a simple task for Group A people to release their purse strings. The bankbook is a source of joy and comfort. Money, they feel, exists to reassure their existence. From it, they derive strength and a purpose for living. In other words, it is not what money can do, but rather what money has done.

Regis Philbin, the television talk show host, has mentioned, perhaps in jest, that "the poorhouse is just around the corner." This "depression days" mentality may still influence Group A and negate their ability to untie the purse strings.

How, then, can Group A people be influenced to share their good fortune and bulging purse with family members in Group C, who are facing economic hardships. Likewise, can Group A people who are penny-pinching without reason be influenced to adopt a different attitude regarding self-indulgence and pampering.

Extricating oneself from a firmly held belief that money is a driving force influencing all aspects of a person's life is not an easy task. There is no magic pill—or chemo—for frugality. Closed-handedness, scrimping, and begrudging themselves the luxuries of life have become firmly implanted in the minds of many Group A people.

The answer lies in the disease itself. Cancer awakens within the individual a spirit of generosity—a realization that days are in short supply, and indeed life is fragile. For some people, "buying a cure" or making amends for past transgressions will extend their lives.

Hugs and kisses are not meant for the lawyer, but rather for the individual who has radically changed his or her lifestyle.

STRATEGIES FOR GROUP A

1. *Gifts for special occasions:* Remember to send checks to recognize birthdays, anniversaries, engagements, and graduations.
2. *Make your presence felt:* Cancer may prevent your appearance at weddings or similar social events. Although your sickness may impose travel restrictions, it does not prevent your sending a generous monetary gift to celebrate.
3. *College tuition:* Sharing the burden of college costs with grandchildren, relatives, or children of friends is quite magnanimous and will be greatly appreciated.
4. *Self-indulgence:* Group A people may have been neglecting their own needs. Now is the time to remove restraints and free yourself from self-denial of life's luxuries. The list of items you can choose from is extensive:

- Taking a cruise
- Taking a land tour
- Buying a new high-definition TV
- Considering a new car
- Hiring a health aide
- Taking a vacation
- Buying new books
- Selecting new clothing
- Eating in fine restaurants
- Subscribing to magazines

Naturally, your oncologist and medical team must be apprised of any travel plans. Your state of health will also influence your self-pampering.

"Releasing Purse Strings" requires disbursement of resources when you are on the surface, not subterranean. Vertical distributions will enhance the memories they encourage—horizontal distributions from your eternal resting place cannot be appreciated with hugs and kisses. That is what you deserve!

END QUOTES

If the rich could hire other people to die for them, the poor could make a wonderful living.

—Jewish proverb

Gentlemen prefer bonds.
—Andrew Mellon

A bank is a place that will lend you money if you can prove that you don't need it.

—Bob Hope

Teach us to give and not to count the cost.
—Ignatius Loyola

It is well to give when asked, but it is better to give unasked, through understanding.

—Kahlil Gibran

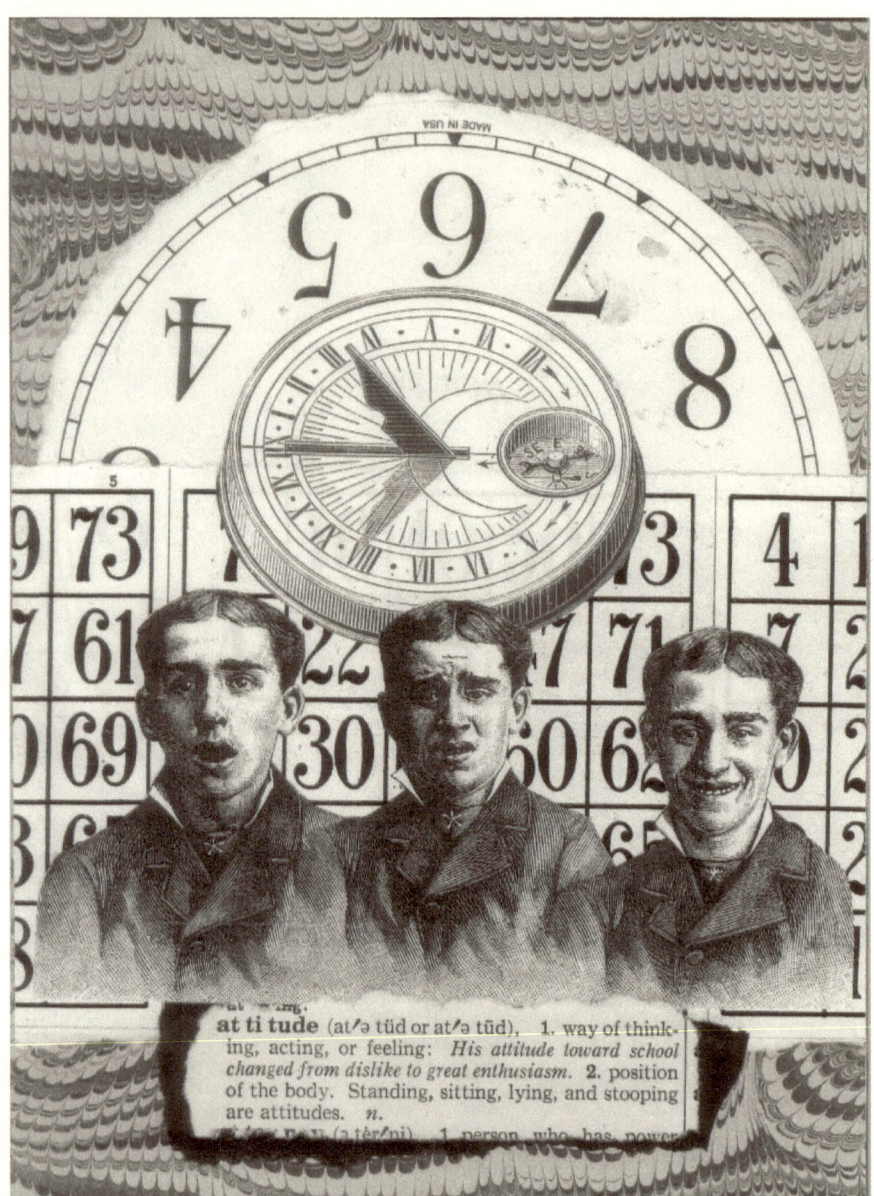

at ti tude (at/ə tūd or at/ə tūd), **1.** way of thinking, acting, or feeling: *His attitude toward school
changed from dislike to great enthusiasm.* **2.** position
of the body. Standing, sitting, lying, and stooping
are attitudes. *n.*

Chapter Twenty-Three

Attitude Adjustment

About the only opinions that do not change are the
ones we have about ourselves.

—Unknown

One of a train engineer's worse nightmares is the possibility of a derailment. Leaving the track staggers the imagination with its capacity to wreak havoc on passengers and cars. "Getting back on track" has become a popular expression meaning that a return to normal conditions has taken place.

A diagnosis of cancer can often lead to a "personality derailment," where the track of positive attitudes has been abandoned, only to be replaced with anger, futility, and depression—not conducive to life support. The wreckage of resentment, hostility, and bitterness created by a diagnosis of cancer are powerful agents of negative forces.

The focus of this chapter delves into the intricacies of attitude. Furthermore, attention will be given to the effect that cancer has on personality and state of mind.

A simple definition of attitude is difficult to present. It consists of:

- Your way of thinking and looking at things
- Your mental outlook
- Your frame of reference
- Your disposition and temperament
- Your level of morale
- Your spiritual climate and the quality of your opinions
- Your relationship to friends and supporters

An attitude "derailment" occurs when cancer alters your personality and your state of mind. You become suspended in an atmosphere of divine discontent. A spirit of sourness pervades your body and makes rosy expectations difficult to achieve. This is not a positive state in which to be. The vitality of hope feeds on invigorating spirits.

Resentment fostered by a diagnosis of cancer fosters a high level of irritation. When this is turned inward, it becomes a gnawing ulcer of the mind. English playwright John Dryden called jealousy and envy "the jaundice of the soul." Cancer patients must ask themselves if they envy the unafflicted and are jealous of the population enjoying good health. The answer may be disturbing to some.

THE MASK

In ancient times, the dramatis personae, or characters in a play, wore masks to portray various roles. The mask was known as a *persona,* or covering for the face. Each of our personalities reflects the mask, unseen, that identifies our attitudes, beliefs, and temperament. There are times that our views become constrictive and cramped because of intolerant behavior and narrow-mindedness. Walking around with a backpack of animosity is a self-destructive attitude. Hostility and abruptness become the mask and complete the derailment from precancerous times.

ANGER

Anger is the response most often expressed when the diagnosis of cancer is disclosed. This primal energy lashes out in all directions and consumes the patient as well. Anger is an attitude-altering agent, and in its fury, it produces negative vibes unfavorable for recovery. It is useless and futile and only creates ill will and antagonism.

Do cancer patients have the right to be angry? Before the question can be answered, several areas should be explored:

At whom am I directing my anger?

Is the anger directed inward—internally—for allowing this to happen?

Think about it. Do you become angry every time you discover that your lottery ticket is not a winner? The anger subsides when hope replaces it; perhaps there will be a winning ticket next time. For some people, it is the luck of the draw. An unfortunate event has happened, and steps must be taken to repair the derailment.

Isn't one illness enough? Deep anger festers subcutaneously and pollutes the soul. Anger inflicts strain on the nervous system and impairs the ability to maintain a healthy attitude. Anger is lethal! It is to be used with caution and discretion—or not at all. Anger is controllable. Losing control is a sign of weakness and poor judgment, qualities not recommended for a speedy recovery. Remember that anger is *danger*ous, toxic to the soul.

DEPRESSION

Hope is a medication! Confidence is chemo for the spirit. Renewed faith strengthens the determination to survive. As hope and faith become diluted, the chances of remission and total cure become obscured.

There is no doubt that pain and suffering are agents of despair. Pain contributes to loss of the life force, and despondency rapidly overtakes the will to survive. Pessimism pervades the psyche, and defeatism yields to despair.

A diagnosis of cancer has the potential of becoming the fence that shuts others out and shuts the patient in. The disease becomes an extinguisher of the sparks of the spirit. This vital energy is needed to prevent the body from sinking into despair and, ultimately, depression.

When life becomes meaningless and hopeless, the prospects for recovery diminish. Depression does not benefit the medical team's plan for recuperation. It burrows into the mind and saps strength from the will to survive.

Be alert to signs of depression. Alienation and a preoccupation with maintaining a distance from loved ones and friends is often an indication. Likewise, withdrawal from routines and indifference to appearance and food can alert the caregiver. Remaining in bed and being unresponsive to pleas from supporters to partake in daily rituals are indicators that all is not well. A visit to your oncologist and medical team is advised for early intervention. Overlooking this behavior is pointless, and it will result in overwhelming despondency. Medical attention is your lifeguard against drowning in a deluge of dejection. Life is a gift! Savor it and reap the benefits of positivism. A healthy mind is the highest peak of a healthy body. Become your own oncologist and supply mental energy to resuscitate your spirit. Fight the doldrums and prosper. To do less is to perpetuate a bleak outlook for the future. Return to life, and life will return to you.

POSITIVE TRANSFERENCE

How can negatives become positives? Can prophets of doom become harmonious with optimists? Questions that must be considered before resistance is altered are quite numerous. Answers are quite thought-provoking. Positive transference—or the expulsion of negative attitudes and replacement with rays of hope—is analogous to a medical protocol. Its importance is of titanic proportions. What remains to be seen is how this interchange can occur when the mind is not cooperative. The oncologist cannot prescribe attitude adjustment in pill or liquid form. Tranquilizers, maybe, but attitudes change from the inside, not the outside.

Positive transference is an exchange of wills— by focusing on the past and recalling days of contentment, the will to survive replaces the will to exist.

The past can be reconstructed and a healthy mental outlook can be achieved by substituting images of bygone times for images of gloomy outlook. See the mind as a picture-making mechanism, with the capability of blocking out adversity in favor of scenes that soothe and comfort. Positive transference has taken place when the desire to live creates a smile on your face, depression fades away, and attitudes improve.

BACK ON TRACK

This final chapter in this survival guide for cancer patients began with an allusion to a train derailment. Getting back on track is a golden rule for recovery that starts from the top, down. That expression of hope will complement your treatments and medications.

Combativeness, bitterness, and hostility have no part in the recovery process. It is up to the individual to restore harmony in the body.

The Siberian tiger, the condor, and the American bald eagle are on the endangered species list. Are you on the list too? Your presence on any list that augurs slim chances for survival must serve as a wake-up call. Hear the trumpets playing Verdi's "Grand Triumphal March" from the opera *Aida*. They are playing it for you and every cancer patient struggling for survival.

Get in line and join the parade. You know what to do!

END QUOTES

The greatest discovery of my generation is that a human being can alter his life by altering his attitude.

—William James

Change starts when someone sees the next step.

—William Drayton

Change is not made without inconvenience, even from worse to better.

—Samuel Johnson

Some people continue to change jobs, mates, and friends—but never think of changing themselves.

—Unknown

Our dilemma is that we hate change and love it at the same time; what we really want is for things to remain the same but get better.

—Sydney J. Harris

Chapter Twenty-Four

Resource Guide

PART I This alphabetical listing of organizations offers information and support services.

1. American Cancer Society
   800-227-2345   www.cancer.org
2. Cancer and Careers
   www.cancerandcareers.org
3. Cancer Care
   800-813-4673   www.cancercare.org
4. Gilda's Club
   888-445-3248   www.gildasclub.org
5. Lance Armstrong Foundation
   512-236-8820   www.livestrong.org
6. National Cancer Institute
   800-422-6237   www.cancer.gov
7. National Coalition for Cancer Survivorship
   877-622-7937   www.canceradvocacy.org
8. Patient Advocate Foundation
   800-532-5274   www.patientadvocate.org
9. People Living with Cancer
   703-797-1914   www.plwc.org
10. Planet Cancer
    www.planetcancer.org
11. Wellness Community
    888-793-9355   www.thewellnesscommunity.org

PART II This alphabetical listing of organizations provides services for specific types of cancer.

1. **Bladder Cancer**
    Bladder Cancer Network
    301-469-6865   www.bcan.org
2. **Brain Tumors**
    American Brain Tumor Association
    800-886-2282   www.abta.org
    National Brain Tumor Foundation
    800-934-2873   www.braintumor.org
3. **Breast Cancer**
    Sisters Network
    866-781-1808   www.sistersnetworkinc.org
    Susan G. Komen Breast Cancer Foundation
    800-462-9273   www.komen.org
    Y-ME National Breast Cancer Org.
    800-221-2141   www.yme.org
4. **Colorectal Cancer**
    Colon Cancer Alliance
    877-422-2030   www.ccalliance.org
5. **Esophageal Cancer**
    Esophageal Cancer Awareness Association
    866-730-3222   www.ECaware.org
6. **Kidney Cancer**
    Kidney Cancer Association
    800-850-9132   www.kidneycancerassoc.org
7. **Leukemia/Lymphoma/Myeloma**
    Leukemia and Lymphoma Society
    800-955-4572   www.lls.org
    Multiple Myeloma Foundation
    203-972-1250   www.multiplemyeloma.org
8. **Bone Marrow Cancer**
    National Marrow Donor Program
    800-627-7692
9. **Lung Cancer**
    Lung Cancer Alliance
    800-298-2436   www.lungcanceralliance.org
    It's Time to Focus on Lung Cancer
    877-646-5864   www.lungcancer.org

10. **Ovarian Cancer**
    Ovarian Cancer National Alliance
    202-331-1332   www.ovariancancer.org
11. **Pancreatic Cancer**
    Pancreatic Cancer Action Network
    877-272-6226   www.pancan.org
12. **Prostate Cancer**
    National Prostate Cancer Coalition
    www.4npcc.org

PART III University-Sponsored Organizations

1. University of Alabama at Birmingham
2. Duke University Cancer Center at Durham, North Carolina
3. University of South Florida Cancer Center at Tampa, Florida
4. University of Michigan Cancer Center at Ann Arbor, Michigan
5. New York University Cancer Institute at New York City, New York
6. Ohio State University Research Institute at Columbus, Ohio
7. Northwestern University Cancer Center at Chicago, Illinois
8. University of Texas Cancer Center at Houston, Texas
9. University of Tennessee Cancer Institute at Memphis, Tennessee
10. University of Utah Cancer Institute at Salt Lake City, Utah
11. Vanderbilt University—Ingram Cancer Center at Nashville, Tennessee

PART IV Clinical Trials

Clinical trials feature experimental treatments and/or drugs offered by pharmaceutical companies and oncologists.

These trials are administered in early-phase and late-phase sections. Each phase has its own qualifications and restrictions. You may wish to go online and contact www.curetoday.com/toolbox for addition information. Naturally, your oncologist is your prime advisor for clinical trials.

The degree to which you utilize any of the resources represented in this chapter depends on the effort you are able to put forth. Resources are meant to serve as a stockpile of information. They definitely come in handy when you are in need of additional knowledge.

Bibliography

Bartlett, John. *Bartlett's Words to Live By.* New York: Little, Brown, & Co., 2006.

Byrne, Robert. *The 2,548 Best Things Anybody Ever Said.* New York: Simon & Shuster, 1982.

Canuth, Gorton. *The Giant Book of American Quotations.* New York: Gramercy Books, 1988.

Cook, John. *The Book of Positive Quotations.* Minneapolis: Fairview Press, 1993.

Fitzhenry, Robert. *Harper Book of Quotations.* New York: Harper-Collins, 1993.

McKenzie, E.C. *14,000 Quips & Quotes.* New York:Wings Books, 1980.

Ratcliffe, Susan. *Little Oxford Dictionary of Quotations.* New York: Oxford Univer. Press, 2005.

Reader's Digest Association. *Quotable Quotes.* New York: Reader's Digest Press, 1997.

Rostand, Edmond. *Cyrano de Bergerac.* New York: Bantam Books, 1951.

Afterword

Charles Dickens, well-known author of *A Christmas Carol,* featuring Ebenezer Scrooge and Tiny Tim, wrote ten lines in *A Tale of Two Cities,* a novel recalling the French Revolution. The words he used are quite representative of the cancer patient's struggle for survival:

> *It was the best of times.*
> *It was the worst of times.*
> *It was the age of reason.*
> *It was the age of foolishness.*
> *It was the epoch of belief.*
> *It was the epoch of incredulity.*
> *It was the season of light.*
> *It was the season of darkness.*
> *It was the spring of hope.*
> *It was the winter of despair.*

Despair or hope—the decision is yours.

www.ingramcontent.com/pod-product-compliance
Lightning Source LLC
Chambersburg PA
CBHW031324290526
45784CB00014B/1111